Pain-Free Living for Drug-Free People

Pain-Free Living for Drug-Free People

A Guide to Pain Management in Recovery

Marvin D. Seppala, M.D.

and

David P. Martin, M.D., Ph.D.

with Joseph Moriarity

HAZELDEN

Hazelden
Center City, Minnesota 55012-0176

1-800-328-0094
1-651-213-4590 (Fax)
www.hazelden.org
All personal stories found in this book were created by the authors to represent
the common experiences of individuals who have dealt with taking prescription medication to relieve pain. Any resemblance to a specific person, living or
dead, or to a specific event is coincidental. This book is not intended as a substitute for the medical advice of physicians. The reader should consult a physician in matters relating to his or her health.

Library of Congress Cataloging-in-Publication Data

Seppala, Marvin D.
    Pain-free living for drug-free people: a guide to pain management in
recovery / Marvin D. Seppala and David P. Martin; with Joseph Moriarity
        p.   cm.
    ISBN-13: 978-1-59285-097-6
    ISBN-10: 1-59285-097-9
    1. Recovering addicts—Health. 2. Substance abuse—Treatment.
    3. Pain—Treatment. I. Martin, David P., 1964–. II. Moriarity, Joseph.
    III. Title.
    RC564.29.S47 2005
    616.86'06—dc22

                                                        2005046394

09   6 5 4 3 2
Cover design by David Spohn
Interior design by Wendy Holdman
Typesetting by Stanton Publications, Inc.

CONTENTS

Introduction

Kathleen's Story

The pain in her tooth had been getting worse by the day. Her jaw was aching, and she was having trouble sleeping. Aspirin and ibuprofen weren't helping nearly enough. She finally had to face the fact that she really did need to go to the dentist to have the tooth examined.

From her dentist, Kathleen learned that the problem would require minor oral surgery. "I can certainly use lidocaine to keep you pain free during the surgery," her dentist told her, referring to a local anesthetic. "But you're going to be pretty sore for at least a day or two, so I'm going to prescribe a painkiller for the first two days. Most of my patients do very well with a combination of acetaminophen and hydrocodone (Vicodin). Fill the prescription before you come in, so you have it ready."

Kathleen had been in recovery from alcoholism for thirteen years and had never relapsed. "And I'm not about to now, either," she told herself. Kathleen was very proud of being chemical free. She was afraid of using anything like hydrocodone. She knew a woman in one of her Twelve Step meetings who'd been addicted to that drug, so she wasn't about to take any chances. "Besides," she told herself, "I've been through a lot. The pain can't be that bad, and the dentist said it would only hurt for a day, two at the most. I can tough it out." She didn't fill the prescription.

Kathleen's surgery was in the late afternoon. On her way home from the dentist's office, she felt wonderful. The dentist had been right; she hadn't felt a thing, and now the tooth problem was resolved.

In the early evening, however, her medication began to wear off. Kathleen's jaw began to hurt. It was pretty sore, but nothing she couldn't get through. "This isn't so bad," she said to herself.

An hour later, the pain was still worsening. Her jaw was pounding, and the pain was jabbing into her head. By eleven o'clock Kathleen was in serious pain, and she didn't know what to do. It was far, far worse than she ever imagined it would be, and it was still intensifying. Kathleen was scared. She actually wished now that she'd filled the dentist's prescription, but it was too late. And besides, she'd thrown out the prescription sheet, thinking at the time that there was no need to have temptation around.

By midnight, Kathleen was desperate. Finally, she jumped into her car and sped off to a neighborhood bar. She ran in, threw down a twenty-dollar bill, and ordered shots until the pain was gone. "I just had to do something to get rid of the pain," she said later. "It hurt worse than anything I'd imagined, and I just didn't know what else to do."

Jake's Story

After fifty-seven very active years, Jake finally had to admit that some of his "parts" were showing signs of wear and tear—specifically his right knee. Jake was a fine athlete and had played a variety of sports for many years: volleyball, racquetball, basketball, and tennis. He also loved in-line skating and skiing. Over time, however, the cartilage in his right knee had become torn and worn down. The result? Chronic knee pain that was continuing to worsen. Jake had done a lot to try to slow the degeneration in his knee. He'd seen a massage therapist regularly and taken up yoga. Both helped keep his muscles strong and flexible, which seemed to lessen his pain. He'd found ibuprofen helped with swelling and pain, but he was worried about using it too much because his doctor told him that it could harm his stomach. He carefully avoided any prescription medicines for pain control. Because Jake had been in recovery from alcohol and drug addiction for more than twenty-five years, he decided to discuss the issue of pain control and relapse in depth with his family doctor.

Because of Jake's increased knee pain, his family doctor recommended that he see an orthopedist, who in turn gave him the unfortunate news that he needed a knee replacement. Jake decided to go ahead with the surgery. Beforehand, however, he set up a meeting with both doctors to discuss pain control for surgery and for his rehab. "I wanted to have everything out in the open," said Jake. "I'd heard that the first couple weeks can be tough. Other people I know needed to use morphine right after surgery and Percocet for the first week or so of rehabilitation. But Percocet contains oxycodone, and I didn't know if I'd dare do that, given my history of addiction. Still, I didn't want to be in agony, either."

Together, the three of them laid out a plan. "The doctors told me I'd be using a morphine pump that I could control right after surgery. That really scared me at first, but both docs assured me that in this case, the only thing I'd feel would be pain relief, not a high. And that was exactly true."

As part of this plan, Jake and his doctors also drew up an agreement that carefully spelled out how he would use prescription medicines after surgery to control his pain, and how his use could be monitored to ensure that he wouldn't trigger his old addiction. His surgery recovery plan also included a number of complementary medicine therapies that he'd had positive experiences with in the past: massage therapy in addition to the physical therapy he'd be receiving; acupuncture to help control pain and rebalance the body's vital energy, or "qi"; and meditation to enhance relaxation and stress reduction.

Jake also felt the need to talk about his upcoming surgery with his sponsor and his recovery-meeting group members. He told everyone why he needed surgery and outlined his plan for controlling pain. "I was nervous about using prescription painkillers because I knew there were some people in my meeting who think that you should never ever use them, no matter the reason," he said. "But my doctors really understood the issues. They said that I wasn't the first person in recovery to have a knee replacement and that if we follow the plan we made, I'd be okay."

Jake's surgery went well. "It did hurt pretty badly right after surgery," said Jake. "Worse than I thought it would, actually. But the morphine worked really well. It didn't trigger any of my addictive patterns, although once I felt a little lightheaded, and I was *really* glad I had something strong like that to use. The first couple weeks of therapy were tough, too. When they take apart your knee and put it back together again, well, I guess you should expect some pain. But the oxycodone helped a lot, and I really feel the complementary therapies made a big difference as well. It's been six weeks now, and things are much better. I'm still doing physical therapy, but I can manage with just ibuprofen now. I got through everything without endangering my recovery, and I hope to be getting back to all my favorite activities again soon. I went back to my meeting, of course, and let everyone know how things went. I think it was good for them to hear that it's possible to go through an operation like I did, and even to use strong painkillers, without messing up your recovery. I think they were pretty surprised, actually."

How to Deal with Pain

It's inevitable, inescapable. Each of us will have to deal with pain that requires medical intervention at some time in our lives, be it acute or chronic. The question we must address, then, is how do we deal with it when it arrives? It is a challenge for all of us, but people who are or were addicted to alcohol or other drugs face a special challenge because some pain medications are addictive. And under certain circumstances, they can trigger relapse. We have written this book precisely to address the issue of pain and pain control for people who are or have been chemically dependent and for their supporting family and friends.

You may have never experienced acute or chronic pain. You might be thinking that it is an issue you'll deal with when the need arises. That is your choice.

We urge you, however, to make a different choice; as the saying goes, "Forewarned is forearmed." Even if you're fortunate enough to be healthy and pain free now, at some point you will have to deal with pain. Jake's and Kathleen's stories illustrate these options clearly. Jake was nervous about his surgery and rehabilitation, so he chose to prepare carefully for his surgery and post-operative pain. He also sought support from his recovery community. As a result, he encountered no problems, despite needing and using prescription pain medications. Yes, it is possible for recovering alcoholics and addicts to use these drugs safely. They shouldn't be the first choice, of course, but with care, they can be used safely.

Kathleen, however, made a different choice. She was nervous, too, about using an addictive drug for pain control, but she made the inaccurate assumption that she could handle everything herself. Her recognition of the potential danger for relapse also showed in her decision not to fill her pain prescription, or even keep her doctor's prescription order. Furthermore, she never really asked her dentist how bad the pain could get. She didn't talk to her sponsor or people at her Twelve Step meeting. And when the pain finally became intolerable, she was unable to see any alternative other than to drink.

Remember, too, that you could find yourself thrust into a situation that requires pain control unexpectedly. You could be in an auto accident, for example, or develop an acute illness. We hope that you will have taken this book's advice and made some preparations for such an occurrence—or that you will think to turn to it for help and use the tools it offers.

It's not unusual for people in recovery to fear using medications, especially ones that can be addictive, even if their drug of choice was solely alcohol. That's sensible and understandable, actually. This book will give you the information you need to address those fears and show you how to take positive, effective steps to deal with both acute and chronic pain without triggering addiction or relapse. You do have options, more than you might guess. While prescription painkillers can be effective for dealing with pain, other medications and therapies, including complementary medicine, are available, especially for chronic pain.

As you begin to explore all the options open to you, this book can help you navigate what probably seems like a confusing maze of medications and therapies. We don't want you ever to find yourself in circumstances as desperate as Kathleen's, in which you feel your only choice is to buy a bottle of whiskey or beg some prescription drugs from a neighbor.

If you are not suffering from acute or chronic pain now, we want you to be prepared—or at least to have an outline of a plan that lays out the steps you will take when the need arises. If you are currently dealing with chronic pain, this book can give you the information you need to develop a more comprehensive plan for managing it.

You don't need to read this book cover to cover; the index can help you find the sections you need. However, reading it cover to cover at some point will give you an excellent overview of this important area of health.

Take Control of Your Health Care

You are ultimately the person who has the final say in your medical care. The better informed you are, the better decisions you can make. And that's true whether you're deciding about conventional or complementary medicine.

As we will stress throughout this book, you will fare much

better if you take some responsibility for your progress and for your health care as a whole. We know that when patients are well informed about their care—when they become partners with the medical staff who are helping them—they achieve better results and are more satisfied with their care.

Certainly, approaches to this task differ, but just taking responsibility for it is a very positive step. Again, we encourage you to be a motivated and well-educated patient in pursuing whatever therapies you choose to help you achieve your goal of pain management without risk of addiction or relapse.

If you simply leave these decisions to your doctor, your family or friends, or any person who gives you recommendations, you may not make the wisest choices. It is only by taking on the responsibility of evaluating your own progress that you will be able to make appropriate decisions about your care.

CHAPTER 1

What Is Pain?

Pain. We've all experienced it many times in our lives. As children, we skinned our knees and elbows, smacked our heads against various objects, fell off bikes and down stairs and off swing sets. And then there were stomachaches, headaches, earaches, sprains—and maybe even a broken bone.

Pain is with us from birth to death. Almost half of all Americans visit doctors and other health care providers to seek treatment and relief from pain each year—7 million of them for newly diagnosed back pain.

Chronic pain is one of America's most costly health problems. Estimated annual costs, including direct medical expenses, lost income, lost productivity, compensation payments, and legal charges, are about $90 billion for back pain alone. To put these expenses in perspective, the total $90 billion spent in 1998 represented 1 percent of the U.S. gross domestic product (GDP), and the $26 billion in direct back pain costs accounted for 2.5 percent of all health care expenditures for that year.[1]

What's more, the cost of chronic pain reaches far beyond financial considerations. For chronic pain sufferers, the cost in quality of life is very high: many are less able or unable to walk or exercise, enjoy natural sleep, perform household chores, attend social activities, drive a car, or have sexual relations. The effect of pain on these people's lives is such that many report that their relationships with family and friends are strained or broken. Following are some examples.

Back pain. Pain in the lower back is one of the most significant pain-related health problems.

- In 1998, 25.9 million Americans reported suffering from back pain.
- Back pain is the most frequent cause of activity limitation in people younger than forty-five years old.
- Thirty-one million Americans are struggling with lower back pain at any given time.
- One-half of all working Americans have back symptoms each year.
- One-third of all Americans over age eighteen had a back problem in the previous five years that was severe enough for them to seek professional help.
- The cost of this care is estimated to be a staggering $50 billion a year—and that's just for the more easily identified costs.[2]

Headaches. According to the National Institute of Neurological Disorders and Stroke (NINDS), as many as 45 million Americans have chronic, severe headaches that can be disabling. Each year people spend more than $4 billion on over-the-counter pain medications for headaches. Migraine sufferers lose more than 157 million workdays annually because of headache pain.[3]

Cancer pain. The majority of patients in intermediate or advanced stages of cancer suffer moderate to severe pain. More than 1.4 million new cases of cancer are diagnosed each year in the United States.[4]

Although we are all familiar with pain, it nevertheless remains a curious, even mysterious, phenomenon. Two people walk through a doorway, for example, and each knocks an elbow against the door frame. One grabs his elbow and cringes; the other barely acknowledges the bump. Why did virtually the same experience result in searing pain in one case and barely noticeable discomfort in the other? Is one person a "crybaby" and the other just being "macho"? Did that similar bump actually register differently in each of them? If so, why? Do they have different attitudes about pain, and if so, would that make a difference?

Pain is universal. The degree to which we feel pain and how we react to it, however, is the result of our own individual biological, psychological, and cultural makeup. Past experience with injuries or illness can influence our sensitivity to pain. Simply stated, pain varies from one person to another, and this varied response also makes it difficult to describe.

A Medical Definition of Pain

As familiar as we all are with pain, can we actually define it? Just what is pain? The accepted medical definition of pain is "an unpleasant sensory and emotional experience associated with actual or potential tissue damage or described in terms of such damage."[5]

Yes, that's a bit dry, but it contains the gist of what we are all familiar with: pain is an unpleasant sensory experience.

The feeling of pain varies enormously, and as a result we use many different words to describe it: *nagging, tingling, dull, sharp, jabbing, burning, pounding,* and *stinging,* to name just a few. Pain ranges from barely noticeable to excruciating. Severe pain can incapacitate a person. Where pain is located in your body can make a difference in its effect. Severe lower back pain, for example, can hamper mobility and may be perceived as much worse than a burn or a cut on your hand.

But there's much, much more to pain when we look deeper. Pain is a sensation we feel—what we usually call the "ouch." It is also an emotional experience, with frustration, anger, sadness, and other feelings often accompanying it.

The definition also acknowledges "actual or potential tissue damage." A broken bone or a burn causes pain that's clearly associated with actual tissue damage. But it is also possible to feel pain even when no true tissue damage is present— a mild burn will hurt despite the fact that you may not have actually damaged your skin.

If you break a bone in your arm, you may experience a rapid heartbeat, sweating, and elevated blood pressure—what seem to be objective signs. However, we know now that those autonomic (or involuntary) responses are not universal, and over time, even with continued pain or tissue damage related to the fracture, those responses can and do, in many cases, return to normal.

So we cannot use elevated blood pressure or increased heart rate as a way to measure pain. Nor can we use X-rays. It's not unusual to see examples of physical abnormalities that aren't painful for everyone. A person may have a slipped disk, an abnormal spine, or advanced arthritis in a joint, for example, yet be living pain free. Conversely, people with no physical evidence of spinal problems may nevertheless expe-

rience back pain. Nor is it unusual for doctors to see a disso-
ciation between objective changes in test results or X-rays,
for example, and the perception of pain. You can have one
without the other.

Finally, pain can be an unpleasant sensory and emotional
experience that is *described* in terms of tissue damage. In other
words, if a person reports that "I have a burning, tearing sensation in my back," then by definition there is pain. He or she
uses those terms to describe the sensation, *even though* there
may not be any observable tissue damage in the back. It may
be difficult to understand, but in such cases, we have to accept a subjective manifestation of pain.

How and why we experience pain is exceedingly complex,
and it can vary widely from person to person. This medical
reality lies at the root of much frustration for people with
chronic pain. Many have had the experience of going to a doctor for their pain and hearing such statements as "Well, you
shouldn't feel pain" or "The X-rays look pretty normal so I can
see no real reason for your pain" or "According to your test
results, there's really nothing wrong with you." Again, difficult though it may be for some doctors—and for people with
chronic pain—to accept, the truth is simply that if something
hurts, then yes, you have real pain.

The Purpose of Pain

Most people consider pain to be a negative experience. For the
majority of people most of the time, however, pain serves a useful purpose: it is a protective warning and a means to help us
avoid injury. What happens, for example, if you accidentally
touch a hot stove burner? You'll *very* rapidly jerk your arm
back without even thinking about it. This reflex is extremely

useful because it helps you avoid injury. Some disorders, such as diabetes, cause people to lose the ability to feel pain. Diabetic patients can experience a degeneration of pain-sensing nerves in their feet, and they no longer recognize when their footwear fits improperly or when a stone is stuck in their shoe. As a consequence, they develop sores that can be very slow to heal.

Pain also helps us know when we have injured ourselves. Let's say you turn your ankle playing basketball. It hurts like crazy to put any weight on it, and because of that burning pain, you leave the game and sit down. Soon you're doing everything you should do to help that injury heal. You're immobilizing and protecting the ankle. If you hadn't felt pain, you might have continued playing, worsening the injury and causing serious, long-term damage to your ankle.

But other pain, such as the daily ache of a migraine or arthritis, doesn't seem to serve any useful purpose. In addition, its constant presence can wear a person down physically, emotionally, and psychologically.

When pain becomes such a problem that it interferes with life's work and normal activities, a person may become the victim of a vicious cycle. Pain may cause a person to become preoccupied with physical symptoms, depressed, and irritable. Depression and irritability often lead to insomnia and weariness, leading to more irritability, depression, and pain. This state is a "terrible triad" of suffering, sleeplessness, and sadness. The urge to stop the pain can make some people drug-dependent and may drive others to have repeated surgeries or resort to questionable treatments. Adding to the problem, this situation can often be as hard on the family as it is on the person suffering from the pain.

We react differently to "familiar" and "unfamiliar" pain.

By the time we're adults, we've all experienced minor burns, stomachaches, and a sprain or two. But how does a middle-aged man react when he suddenly feels a crushing pressure in his chest after a big meal? He may tell himself it's just indigestion, but he'll also wonder if he's having a heart attack. It's certainly a warning that something's wrong, but the cause is not so obvious—it's not a burn or a twisted ankle. The pain will still likely protect him from harm because he'll probably go to an emergency room for tests to see what's happening. If the pain continues, he'll probably be frightened and worried—the emotional aspect of pain. Should you twist your ankle, you might feel a little frustrated, but you'd quickly accept the situation. If, however, you fear you're having a heart attack or that you might have cancer, the emotional aspect of pain can cause you to suffer tremendously. Conversely, women can experience excruciating pain during childbirth, but rarely do they complain about it later. They may acknowledge that it was bad for a while, but it's usually quickly forgotten and has very few long-term consequences, despite its severity. The context and meaning of your pain have much to do with your perception of it.

Pain is a very personal experience that grows out of a particular context or situation and is heavily influenced by a person's prior encounters with it. Childhood experiences, how you've seen your family and friends react to pain, and your culture's attitude toward pain all affect the way you react to it.

The Biology of Pain

With a basic understanding of how our bodies process sensory information, we can better appreciate how we actually experience pain, and we can better see why treating chronic pain can be such a challenge at times. Let's begin with the function of the nervous system.

Our nervous system is made up of two primary parts: the *central nervous system,* which includes the brain and spinal cord, and the *peripheral nervous system,* which extends from our spinal cord to our skin, muscles, and internal organs. In brief, pain results from a series of electrical and chemical communications involving the peripheral nerves, the spinal cord, and the brain. Let's look more closely at this process.

The Peripheral Nervous System

The peripheral nervous system contains three types of nerves:

- *Autonomic nerves* have the job of maintaining normal body functions such as heart rate, blood pressure, digestion, and sweating.
- *Motor nerves* allow us to carry out muscle movements at all levels: walking, lifting, sitting, using eating utensils, and so on.
- *Sensory nerves* let us perceive our world—to feel the chair we sit on, the book we hold, the clothes we wear—and they are the nerves that let us feel pain, too.

The sensory nerves are a vast network of fibers branching throughout our body. This array of specialized nerves is designed to sense certain aspects of the environment, such as temperature, pressure, and touch. Under mild stimulation, we feel warmth or coolness. The tendons and ligaments that move our joints have sensors that note how far a given joint is moving and how hard the muscle is pulling. These sensations help us judge our position in space and tell us, for example, how forcefully to lift an object. When those tendons and ligaments are pulled to extremes—turning an ankle or bending a joint farther than it's supposed to go, for example—we feel pain.

In addition to these sensory nerve endings, we also have other nerve endings called *nociceptors* that detect actual or potential tissue damage. Nociceptors are sensitive to particular chemical substances that are released when tissues are injured. Collectively, these fibers are nonspecialized injury sensors (*noci* means "injury" in Latin).

We have millions of nociceptors in our skin, bones, joints, and muscles and in the protective membranes around our internal organs. Nociceptors are concentrated in areas where we're more likely to be injured, such as our fingers and toes. That's why a sliver in your finger hurts more than one in your leg or arm. In fact, you might not even feel a sliver in the latter locations. There can be as many as 1,300 nociceptors in just one square inch of skin. Our muscles, which lie protected beneath our skin, have fewer nociceptors. Our internal organs, which are further protected by bones and muscle, have even fewer still.

When nociceptors pick up a harmful stimulus, they send their pain messages in the form of electrical impulses along a peripheral nerve to the spinal cord and brain. But the amount of signaling is not always the same. Nociceptors can become "revved up" or "sensitized."

Inflammation and Peripheral Sensitization

Inflammation is the body's response to tissue injury or an infection, and it's actually the body's way of initiating healing. More blood flows to the damaged area, and it is seen as redness and swelling. An inflamed area feels warm to the touch because of the extra blood flow. The classic terms for describing inflammation are *rubor, tubor, calor,* and *dolor,* the Latin terms for "redness," "swelling," "heat," and "pain."

The area hurts because the chemicals associated with inflammation also sensitize the nociceptors. Now the nociceptors need only a small amount of stimulus to send a pain signal. As a result, your pain threshold is lower. If you've ever had a sunburn, for example, you've noticed that the mere touch of your clothing on your skin hurts. That's sensitization. This sensitization also turns up the volume of the pain signal. Normally, a little bit of stimulus would result in only a little nerve signaling, but now, it results in a lot of nerve signaling. When you have inflammation near nociceptors, they get revved up. This process is called *peripheral sensitization.* It is an example of *neuromodulation*—a way the nervous system changes its responsiveness.

Keep this process in mind as, in later chapters, we refer to the role of inflammation and sensitization in pain control. Anti-inflammatory medications are often used effectively in treating pain.

The Role of the Spinal Cord

Let's return now to the nervous system's process of pain signaling. The spinal cord is the next step for the nerve transmission. Nociceptive information comes from an extremity or from the periphery of the body. Those signals do not, however, go directly to the brain. First, the spinal cord itself does some information processing, and this is the next level of neuromodulation. When pain messages reach your spinal cord, they meet other nerve cells that act as gatekeepers, filtering the pain messages on their way to your brain.

Doctors and scientists once thought that the nerves that transmitted pain were analagous to the electrical wiring in a house, where the circuits are obvious and hardwired. Nerves were seen as simply communicating pain signals from injured or diseased parts of the body to the brain. Thanks to new research, we now know that this system is far more complex. One important new discovery concerns sensitization. Studying this process has opened doors to understanding chronic pain and the reasons it can be disproportionately severe. Simply put, when pain signals are transmitted from injured or diseased tissues, these signals can then activate, or sensitize, pain pathways. This is called *central sensitization,* and it is similar to what happens in the periphery with inflammation.

Pain messages can also decrease as they pass through your spinal cord. Other sensations may overpower and diminish the pain signals. Maybe you injured your foot, but then you massaged or applied pressure to the injured spot. In either case, as a result, the warnings sent by your peripheral nerves are downgraded.

The brain also has nerves going to the spinal cord that can dampen, or "turn down," the sensation of pain. This is a process performed by the endogenous (naturally occurring) opiate system, which creates morphinelike chemicals in the body called *enkephalins* and *endorphins*. When they are released, they attach to special receptors in the brain and spinal cord that stop the pain. Stories of their powerful effect are told periodically in the sports pages. An athlete may rise to incredible levels of performance despite a tissue injury that should have caused severe pain—yet the athlete reports feeling no discomfort. These body chemicals can down-regulate pain signals to allow us to function in spite of the body's messages that we have tissue damage.

Pain Pathways to the Brain

The brain, then, is the final receptor of the pain message. The moment you cut your finger or step on a piece of glass, you don't feel pain because your brain doesn't know about the injury yet. Until the signal reaches the brain, you haven't, by definition, had pain. When pain messages reach your brain, they arrive at the thalamus, a station for sorting and switching located deep inside the brain. The thalamus forwards the pain messages simultaneously to three specialized regions. One pathway goes to the *somatosensory cortex,* the sensory or discriminative part of the brain that lets us locate the pain. The second pathway leads to the brain's emotional center, the *limbic system,* which controls feelings and motivation. The third leads to the *frontal cortex,* the "thinking" part of our brain. Our awareness of pain, therefore, is a complex combination of sensing, feeling, and thinking.

In general, pain signals move fastest along the first pathway. For example, when you bite your tongue, you instantly notice a sharp stab of pain. You know exactly where the pain is and react very quickly by relaxing your bite. Next, a split second later, you experience a sense of anger or displeasure— the emotional part of the pain. These two reactions are distinct and staggered slightly in time because they have traveled to different parts of the brain. These aspects of pain are inseparable, although which of the two reactions becomes more dominant—as well as the intensity of the reactions—depends both on the situation *and* on the person experiencing them.

At the brain level, reaction to pain is very individualized. On one end of the spectrum are people who have dramatic control over their emotions and their brain, often through the practice of meditation or hypnosis. There are yogis, for example, who can sit in a hot box for hours or lie on a bed of nails and seemingly feel no discomfort. On the other end of the continuum are people so nervous and fragile that even the slightest injury throws them off-kilter. They nearly always seem to be debilitated by physical pain and the emotional pain brought on by the challenges of daily life.

It is difficult to explain the broad spectrum of reactions to pain simply based on what's happening in the environment: one person lies on a bed of nails and doesn't complain while another's day is ruined by a sliver. Such differences may be related to pain processing in the periphery and in the spinal cord, but in these extremes, the difference is also likely in the brain. Regardless, these modulations happen at all three levels, and it is most important to note that people differ dramatically in how they react to pain.

The meaning, or significance, of the pain affects how it is perceived. In a carefully controlled experiment, two groups of subjects underwent an identical diagnostic procedure. A small balloon was inflated to the same volume in each person, causing some stretching and discomfort. Both groups were asked to rate how much pain they felt.

With one group, the medical staff made vaguely worrisome comments in front of the patients—statements such as "Does that look all right to you? Does that look like a tumor? I'm not sure. That's a bit strange." In front of the other patients, the examiners made reassuring statements such as "Everything's going fine. That looks perfectly normal. You're doing great."

Even though both sets of patients had exactly the same amount of stretching, the group that heard the worrisome comments rated their pain and discomfort much higher than the group who heard reassuring statements. The only difference was in what they heard and their interpretation of it. Clearly, the mind can have a profound effect on how we experience pain.

Pain Behavior

Behaviorist theory says that it's not possible to really know why people do what they do because we can't ever "get inside" other people's heads. Rather, we can only observe their actions. Pain behavior, then, is anything we say or do that lets another person know or think we're in pain, such as sighing, screaming, crying, limping, clutching an ankle, or using a cane.

Interestingly, pain behavior in a person can be increased, lessened, or even extinguished depending on the actions of others, such as siblings, parents, a spouse, or medical personnel. For example, while walking with his mother, a little boy falls, skins his knee, and breaks into tears. His mother says, "Come on, let's keep going. That's really nothing to cry over." After a bit, the child starts to limp, and the mother says, "Don't be a baby. Stop that. You're not really hurt." Here, the child has received somewhat negative reinforcement for his pain behavior. If he continues to get this kind of reaction, he will learn quite quickly that it's not a good idea to show pain behavior, and as he grows up, he'll likely continue to suppress pain behavior.

On the other hand, let's say that after the boy fell and started to cry, his mother hugged him, brushed the dirt off the scrape, gave it a little kiss, and said, "Oh, dear, that must really hurt. I'm sorry for you. Maybe an ice cream cone will help it feel better." If responses like this continue, the child may soon learn that having pain isn't so bad after all, and there's usually some nice reward as a result.

As we grow older, such interactions happen with employers, spouses, relatives, and friends. Clearly, people's environments and their relationships affect their pain behavior. People learn, either consciously or unconsciously, to react in certain ways to pain. And more important, people's reactions to chronic pain can differ dramatically as a result.

While everyone exhibits pain behavior, pain specialists find that only a small minority actually have a conscious will to take advantage of their pain, to benefit from what is known as "secondary gain." But it does happen. Perhaps someone really hates a job and doesn't want to return to work. Or perhaps the sufferer has the opportunity to make a lot of money in a lawsuit. These may be motivators to accentuate and exaggerate a pain situation.

Today's scientists and doctors realize that pain is not triggered like a light switch—flip it and the "pain" light goes on; something happens that can cause pain, and bingo, we feel it.

Perhaps a more accurate analogy for the body's processing of pain would be a complex system such as a telephone network. Signals flow back and forth through a number of channels. Much switching, noise, and interference take place to amplify the signals or minimize them. Pain is *not* simply an inevitable reflex between what happens to your body and how you feel it. It is both a physiological and a psychological phenomenon that is malleable over time.

CHAPTER 2

Types of Pain

There are three basic ways to differentiate pain, based on its

- *duration:* whether it is acute (short term) or chronic (long term)
- *underlying cause:* whether it is due to an injury (trauma), arthritis, cancer, chemotherapy, or surgery, for example
- *neuroanatomy:* for example, whether it is somatic (coming from the skin, muscle, or bone), visceral (from the internal organs), or neuropathic (from an injury to the nervous system)

Classifying Pain Based on Duration

Acute Pain

Acute pain is usually caused by tissue damage and is the kind that accompanies illness, injury, or surgery. Acute pain may be mild and last just a short time, such as pain from an insect sting or a stubbed toe. Or it can be severe and last for weeks or months, such as pain from a burn, a pulled muscle, or a broken bone. An illness like shingles or the stomach flu can also cause acute pain.

When you have acute pain, you know exactly where it hurts. A headache, a skinned knee, an ankle sprain, and pain from surgery are examples of acute pain. Acute pain usually goes away in a fairly short and predictable period with correct treatment of its underlying cause. The skin on the knee heals, ankle tendons heal and retighten, and the surgical incision closes. In general, any kind of pain that comes from an illness or a trauma and lasts for a short period of time can be termed acute pain.

Chronic Pain

Chronic pain is pain that persists for a long time. Pain is generally described as chronic when it lasts three months or longer. In fact, the word *chronic* actually comes from the Greek word *kronos,* which means "time." Arthritis and back pain are examples of chronic pain.

As with acute pain, chronic pain spans a wide range of sensations and intensity. It can feel aching, pounding, burning, dull, or sharp. The pain may remain constant, or it can come and go, like low back pain.

Unlike those with acute pain, however, chronic pain sufferers may not know why they're in pain at all. The original injury may seem to be completely healed, yet the pain remains and may even have grown worse. Chronic pain can also occur without any indication of injury. Years ago, people who complained of pain that had no apparent cause were thought to be imagining it or simply trying to get attention. We now know that such chronic pain is real.

What other differences are there between the two? Acute pain usually has less effect on a person's long-term outlook, because by definition, it gets better quickly. People with chronic pain, however, face the prospect of living with it over a long period of time.

In addition, while the medicines used to treat acute pain may have side effects, they can be of less concern because the medicines will be used relatively briefly. With chronic pain, however, doctors must be much more careful because a patient may be exposed to a medication long enough for side effects to become a problem.

Classifying Pain Based on Underlying Cause

In the vast majority of cases, it is possible to determine a cause for pain: an injury such as a broken bone, a degenerative condition such as arthritis, or a surgical or dental procedure.

Classifying pain based on its underlying cause is useful because it may allow the use of specific or unique treatments. For example, the pain of rheumatoid arthritis responds to some medications that only work for that disease. Similarly, some surgeries can be performed under regional anesthesia that provides pain control for the specific operation.

In some cases, such as fibromyalgia, there may not be an identifiable abnormality that is the source of the pain. For example, this condition is thought to result from hypersensitivity to pain within the central nervous system—a condition that cannot be detected with scans or blood tests. Nevertheless, making the diagnosis can lead to more effective and specific treatments.

A Special Case: Cancer Pain

When considering pain, most people view cancer-caused pain as a separate category—not because it is by definition worse than pain from other causes, but because it often has a higher degree of psychological impact. (Cancer pain also has some particular medical complexities as well.)

In chapter 1 we described an experiment in which two groups of subjects underwent an identical medical procedure. The group that heard worrisome comments from the staff rated their pain and discomfort much higher than the group who heard reassuring comments.

Imagine, for example, that you hurt your knee playing racquetball and were told by your doctor that you needed surgery to repair torn tissue in the joint. You're also told that the surgery would take only about an hour, that you'd return home the same day, and that you'd be able to resume normal life activities, with some caution, within a few days or weeks. Despite some postsurgery pain and some trouble walking for a few days, you'd probably not be worried. The psychological aspects of your pain would likely be minimal because you understand that pain can usually be expected to go away as the body heals. Or perhaps you have chronic pain in your back. Most people realize that while uncomfortable, back pain is not life-threatening. Despite being chronic, distressing, and even activity-limiting, which certainly can have an emotional effect, this problem will not likely devastate you.

But a diagnosis of cancer, no matter the type, can trigger a whole different range of powerful emotions and reactions. It has a profound psychological impact, not only on the person receiving the diagnosis, but also on his or her family and friends.

Why? Because until fairly recently, most types of cancer were incurable. Although remarkable strides have been made in cancer treatment, when people hear that they have cancer, they still usually assume that they're going to die soon. They have that assumption not only because cancer itself often has been (and still can be) fatal, but also because its treatment implies a series of medical interventions that can be extremely uncomfortable: surgery, some of which can be disfiguring; chemotherapy, which can cause nausea, hair loss, and weakness; and radiation therapy, which can also make a person feel very ill.

Cancer is a life-altering diagnosis. It can be emotionally devastating, too, particularly when it comes to a person in the prime of life or just starting retirement, for example. Suddenly everything is up in the air. Nothing is certain. Hopes and dreams are dashed. Worries about what will happen to a spouse or children can be overwhelming. In contrast, enduring a broken arm or hip surgery or limits on some activities due to chronic pain pales in comparison and rarely has such impact. We distinguish cancer pain as a separate category because of its psychological effect and its association with ongoing treatment that itself may cause pain.

Today, however, many cancers are more treatable than ever before. A diagnosis of cancer is no longer an automatic death sentence. Of course, some cancers still respond poorly to treatment. Many others, however, respond quite well—some so well, in fact, that they can now be regarded more as manageable chronic diseases than as terminal illnesses. Like other chronic problems, cancer can be something with which people simply learn to live.

People in recovery should take caution if they receive a cancer diagnosis; it shouldn't be used as an excuse to ignore the rest of this book's advice. They may very well need to address pain management issues because they may have many years ahead of them. That's time they can and should spend in recovery, not in the throes of addiction.

When, however, patients are near the end stages of a terminal disease, medical staff can justify using more potentially addictive or harmful drugs. At this point, comfort and pain control in a person's final days are more important considerations. Such patients may not suffer any side effects, such as addiction or organ damage, because they won't live long enough for them to appear. A doctor, for example, might use morphine for a person with a history of abuse because many would agree that a relapse in the last day or two of life is justifiable.

Classifying Pain Based on Neuroanatomy

Based on neuroanatomy, there are three types of pain: somatic, visceral, and neuropathic. *Somatic pain* flows from body structures such as the bones, muscles, or skin. It is the most typical kind of pain and is familiar to everyone.

Visceral pain stems from problems with the viscera, the body's internal organs—such as the heart, lungs, intestines, spleen, and so on—but it may be felt in unexpected ways. Why? Because the nociceptors on our organs are not connected to the brain in a way that gives a precise sense of the pain's location. So, for example, if your intestines are distended by gas or a tumor, you might feel cramping or nausea or both. Pain in the heart muscle from a heart attack might be felt in a number of seemingly unrelated places: your left arm, back, or jaw. A woman having a heart attack might only feel extremely nauseated and tired. If your spleen is injured, you're likely to feel pain in your shoulder, and a pancreatic tumor can result in back pain. Visceral pain, then, may be deceptive.

The third type of pain is *neuropathic,* caused by injury to the nervous system itself: nerves, spinal cord, or brain. It may result from an accident, infection, or surgical procedure, but the pain continues after the injury or surgical wounds heal. It is the damaged nerve, not the original injury, that causes neuropathic pain. Once damaged, a nerve can continue to send "incorrect" pain signals. For example, diabetes can damage small nerves in the hands and feet, causing a painful burning sensation in the fingers or toes. Scientists don't completely understand why damaged nerve cells sometimes send pain messages for no reason. One possible explanation is that the ends of damaged nerves grow into a tangle of nerve fibers that fire spontaneously and send pain signals which seem to bypass the checks and balances of the body's normal nervous system.[1]

Defining a person's type of pain is important for deciding what kinds of medications should be used, because somatic, visceral, and neuropathic pain respond to different types of medicines. Combinations of these categories of pain are also possible. A person could have acute or chronic cancer pain, for example. Cancer pain may be somatic, visceral, and neuropathic. Traumatic pain can be acute or chronic.

As you can see, the phenomena encompassed by our single word *pain* are actually very diverse and complex. A basic understanding of the types of pain and how they interact ultimately will help you ask better questions and make more informed decisions when working with doctors to treat pain.

CHAPTER 3

Addiction and Its Treatment

No one takes a first drink of alcohol, snorts a line of cocaine, or smokes a cigarette with the intention of becoming addicted. When first using such drugs, people are simply deciding to do something that makes them feel good. But with continued use, these people can find themselves addicted. They depend on the drug not simply to feel good, but to feel *normal*. Using drugs is no longer a choice; it becomes a necessity. People don't plan to become addicts. In a sense, it just happens.

Alan Leshner, former director of the National Institute on Drug Abuse, calls this the "oops phenomenon." It happens when occasional use of a drug turns into weekly use, then daily use, and eventually into a surprising and disturbing realization: "I'm addicted."[1]

Certain factors, however, can greatly increase the risk of addiction, including genetics, personality, and social/environmental issues such as a childhood history of emotional or physical abuse and exposure and access to drugs. While these nonpharmacological factors do play a role, the effects of alcohol and other drugs on the central nervous system remain the primary cause of drug addiction. Nonpharmacological factors seem to be important in influencing initial drug use and in determining how rapidly an addiction develops. For some substances, nonpharmacological factors may actually interact with the drug's pharmacological action to produce addiction.

Most, if not all, drug users start out using only occasionally, and their use is both voluntary and under their control. But with the passage of time and continued drug use, things change: voluntary use becomes compulsive, that is, users lose control and cannot stop. This occurs because, over time, use of addictive drugs changes the brain. In some cases, it's in dramatic and negative ways; in other cases, it's more subtle. But the change is always destructive. Addiction is characterized by compulsive use of the substance, despite negative consequences.

To really understand the powerlessness over substances that alcoholics and addicts experience, it's helpful to hear one person's story. Though each story is unique, the common themes of denial, manipulation, and continued use despite lost relationships and ruined lives run through them all. Here, Mark tells his story—a story that is at once unique and typical of those addicted to alcohol or other drugs.

Mark's Story

I grew up in Chicago, one of six kids. My dad worked three jobs during most of my childhood, and my mom dedicated her life to taking care of her family. She had anxiety disorders, and it seemed that she didn't have time to think of herself. I don't remember a whole lot of my childhood except that I felt alone and different from the other kids.

After graduating from college, I married a girl I met in school and got a job in the business world. Just a pretty standard story. I do, however, remember being very drunk at the wedding. So drunk, in fact, that I went home with my new wife and passed out for many hours. At the time, that didn't really seem strange.

In my working life, I got "take-out" drinks for the daily train ride home. First, a few beers for the ride, and then after a couple years, the beers turned into martinis. I also had the softball leagues and the Christmas parties, Cubs and Bears games, and, with them all, more and more drinking.

What I see now, without a doubt, is that I was beginning to rot inside. All those things I wanted to be when I grew up— a decent person and a churchgoing family man—were slowly fading into impossibility. I went where alcohol was served and sneaked it in where it wasn't served. Sure, I tried to quit. I knew I was going downhill, but I just couldn't stop.

So I got divorced, remarried, and started all over again. There was a hole inside of me that I couldn't fill. It seemed alcohol would do it for a while, but I kept needing more and more of it to fulfill its purpose.

The mornings would bring great anxiety, depression, and overwhelming feelings of utter despair and hopelessness. So I did what I had trained myself to do: when I felt bad, I drank. Alcohol had become my Higher Power without my having chosen it to be. I couldn't leave it or keep it far from my thoughts for even a short time.

One Friday morning on the way to work, I passed a church sign that I looked at every day, even though I really didn't want to. It said something like "God has not moved from you; you are the one who has moved away from Him." I remember asking God to just leave me alone and let me finish going down this road of destruction.

Perhaps God had heard my unconscious plea for help and saw my undeclared surrender, because I hit bottom the next day without even knowing what that meant. Hadn't I just sat, holding my two-month-old son, and yelled at my wife to take him because I couldn't stand holding him while he cried? Hadn't I just missed my two-year-old daughter's birthday party because I was sitting in the upstairs bedroom drinking a bottle of whiskey while a whole house full of people asked where I was? The end had come. My wife woke up that night, saw I was incoherent from drinking every ounce of alcohol in the house, and sent me to the hospital.

Mark, the college graduate and corporate executive, had obtained a new title: chronic alcoholic. Yes, that's what I was, even though I never got a DUI, was never inside a jail, and had a nice house, two cars, and a good incentive and retirement plan. Chronic alcoholic? Seemed impossible.

In the hospital, I said to my counselor, "Please help me with my problems and then I won't have to drink so much." My counselor responded, "Mark, you have it completely backwards. Quit drinking, and many of your problems will go away."

I attended my first Alcoholics Anonymous meeting at the hospital. I remember all the negative feelings I had as I sat at that meeting, sober and scared: anxious, shaky, and just bad. What I didn't understand was that this state of being had been produced by my alcoholism, which had totally defeated me spiritually, mentally, emotionally, and physically.

This was the beginning of a whole new life for me. In a very real and special way, as has happened to so many others, I was truly born again. Now everything is new. My life in AA is better than it's ever been, even before my first drink. My boy is seven now, and he is the kid I always wanted to be. He's smart, confident, and athletic, and he loves his dad. We hang around together and are building a relationship I could only dream about before I got sober. My little girl hugs me and kisses me and takes such good care of her brother.

I am getting out of life what I always wanted. Not from a stinking bottle, but from a program of honesty and love. The hole I was trying to fill with alcohol is now being filled with a spirit and a joy of life. I still struggle with the normal problems of life. But as long as I stay sober, I have a base to work from. When I was drinking, I was terrified of dying because I knew that I would die a miserable man. But if I die now, I will die sober, happy, and free.

What Is Addiction?

While people in the addiction field have been arguing for decades that addiction to alcohol or other drugs is a disease, it's only relatively recently that research on brain chemistry has made the nature of the disease of addiction much clearer.

Addiction is actually a brain disorder in which the person becomes dependent on a substance because of the effect the substance has on his or her brain. It is the brain's reward system that is primarily involved in addiction. Research has demonstrated that addictive substances cause the release of neurotransmitters such as dopamine, serotonin, GABA (gamma-amino butyric acid), and norepinephrine, which are the brain's own "feel good" chemicals. Over time, the release of these chemicals, triggered by substance use, can alter the workings and sometimes the actual structure of the brain. The addicted person begins to crave the euphoric experiences and prefers them to normal states of reality.

Today, we consider addiction to be a biopsychosocial illness; some would say it's a spiritual illness. We also know that its focal point is located in the brain. The fact is, drug addiction is a *brain disease*. While every type of drug of abuse has its own trigger for affecting or transforming the brain, many of the results of this transformation are strikingly similar regardless of the addictive drug used. The effects that take place in the brain range from fundamental and long-lasting changes in its biochemical makeup to changes in mood and personality, memory processes, and motor skills.

These effects include specific changes in the structure and function of the brain. Thanks to recent advances in research, including magnetic resonance imaging (MRI), positron emission tomography (PET) scans, and computed tomography (CT) scans, we have, literally, a much more complete picture of those changes.

Drugs Change Brain Structure

Using addictive substances causes actual *structural* changes in the human brain. Long-term drinking, for example, shrinks this vital organ. Autopsies consistently show that chronic alcoholics have lighter and smaller brains than nonalcoholics of the same age and gender.

Computerized scanning techniques also reveal how addiction harms or even kills brain cells. Research indicates, for example, that methamphetamine (speed) damages cells that produce dopamine, a chemical in the brain that helps to create feelings of euphoria. Methamphetamine use can even trigger a process called *apoptosis*, in which brain cells actually self-destruct, a process that normally occurs only in very unusual circumstances.

In long-term alcoholics, such changes can be devastating. Studies indicate that 50 to 75 percent of these drinkers show some kind of cognitive decline, even after they detoxify and abstain from alcohol. According to the National Institute on Alcohol Abuse and Alcoholism, alcoholic dementia is the second-leading cause of adult dementia in the United States, exceeded only by Alzheimer's disease.[2]

Drugs Alter Brain Function

The effects of addiction on the brain don't stop with brain size. Research over the past decade reveals that addictive drugs also alter the function of the brain—the very way that cells work.

Human beings are "wired" with *neurons* (nerve cells) that form the brain and spinal cord. Neurons interconnect with one another through junctions called *synapses*. Researchers used to think that neurons passed signals to each other by sending electrical impulses across synapses, similar to electricity jumping the gaps in a car's spark plugs. Today we know that chemicals called *neurotransmitters*—not "sparks"— cross those synapses. The constant exchange of neurotransmitters makes it possible for the brain to send messages through vast chains of neurons to direct our thoughts, feelings, and behavior.

Addictive drugs wreak havoc with this normal exchange of neurotransmitters in many ways. For example, drugs can

- flood the brain with excess neurotransmitters
- stop the brain from making neurotransmitters
- bind to receptors in place of neurotransmitters
- block neurotransmitters from entering or leaving neurons
- empty neurotransmitters from parts of the cells where they're normally stored, causing the neurotransmitters to be destroyed
- increase the number of receptors for certain neurotransmitters
- make some receptors more sensitive to certain neurotransmitters
- make other receptors less sensitive to neurotransmitters, leading to tolerance
- interfere with the reuptake system by preventing neurotransmitters from returning to the sending neuron[3]

A Look at Dopamine

Dopamine is one of the primary neurotransmitters involved in addiction, and it has received special attention from addiction researchers because of its apparent role in mood regulation, motivation, and reward processes. Although there are several dopamine systems in the brain, the *mesolimbic dopamine system* appears to be the most important for motivational processes. All the major drugs of abuse—alcohol, nicotine, opioids, and cocaine—produce their potent effects on behavior by enhancing mesolimbic dopamine activity. In other words, they increase dopamine levels. That's a "good news–bad news" scenario. The good news is that the excess dopamine creates powerful feelings of pleasure, at least temporarily. The bad news is that these excess levels take a long-term toll on brain chemistry and promote addiction.

To understand this concept, remember the biological term *homeostasis,* a word that literally means "same state." With homeostasis, the brain seeks to maintain a constant level of cellular activity. That stable level is critical to regulating our behavior. When supplies of dopamine fluctuate normally, we can experience the ordinary pleasures of life, such as eating and having sex, without the compulsion to seek those pleasures in self-destructive ways.

When consistently subjected to artificially high levels of dopamine from use of a drug, however, the brain "down-shifts" its reaction to this neurotransmitter. The brain comes to depend on the presence of a drug in order to maintain homeostasis and function normally. Thus the "normal" state of the brain now requires the presence of the drug.

That's precisely the problem. If the extra dopamine supplied by drugs is missing, the alcoholic or drug addict feels much less pleasure. In fact, these people instead often experience depression, fatigue, and withdrawal. To the addict, it seems that the only relief from these symptoms is to use more drugs. It all adds up to craving: the addict's constant drive to obtain the chemical of choice.

Drugs Hijack the Brain's Reward Circuit

In addiction, craving for alcohol or other drugs becomes so powerful that it rules the addict's life. This power results in part from changes to a specific path of neurons throughout the brain: the "pleasure system" or "reward circuit." The reward circuit has been studied extensively in rodents, and since biochemical processes in these animals are similar to those of human beings, the results of this research are particularly significant.

In a classic experimental design, researchers attach electrodes to points in the brains of living rodents—locations that correspond to the reward circuit. When rodents press a special lever in their cages, a small electrical current travels via the electrodes directly to the animals' reward circuit. Typically, some of the rodents press the lever compulsively, thousands of times, until they finally collapse in exhaustion.

In another experiment with rats conducted nearly twenty-five years ago, scientists gave thirteen rats access to as much cocaine as they wanted, along with food and water, of course. Within one month, twelve of the thirteen rats had died. The thirteenth died the next week. These animals stopped eating, quit having sex, and suspended their nesting activities. They did nothing but use cocaine—until they simply died of malnutrition and thirst.

Humans and other animals all have what are called "drive states." They include our instincts to eat, sleep, drink, procreate, and have social interaction, but the most basic drive state is simply survival. The power of cocaine caused the rats in this experiment to override the most basic instinct of all: their drive to survive. Humans, sadly, will do the same. For example, drug addicts will unhesitatingly use a needle contaminated with HIV-positive blood, knowing that they are likely to become infected with a fatal disease.

Leshner, the former director of the National Institute on Drug Abuse, uses the term "hijacked brain." This is apt, because an addict is no longer in control of the brain. It's been hijacked by these addictive substances.[4] These findings provide a clue to the power of the reward circuit in human beings, which extends from the midbrain to another section called the *nucleus accumbens*. This region is where drugs of abuse create their effect by masquerading as natural chemicals. Research shows that the nucleus accumbens seems to have a particular role in telling us what might be pleasing or good for us. Drugs like cocaine and amphetamine release remarkably more dopamine into key synapses over a longer period of time in this brain reward pathway than do other normal stimuli, such as great food or sex. These drugs produce an excessive amount of dopamine; therefore, they are incredibly reinforcing. Because they tap directly into a brain circuit that repeats to us, in effect, "Yes, that was good; let's do it again and let's remember exactly how we did it," people will take these drugs again and again and again.

For the person who uses chemicals to repeatedly stimulate the reward circuit, the prospect of abstaining from those chemicals can seem as hopeless and absurd as the idea of abstaining from food. An overpowering drive to drink or use other drugs compromises the user's will, changing what was once a voluntary behavior into an involuntary one. The "normal" state is now only achieved with use of the drug.

Obtaining the drug becomes the top priority in the addict's life. Even everyday emotions such as loneliness can prompt a powerful desire to use substances and attain that high again. External cues, such as certain people, places, and things associated with drug use, can also trigger that desire. These internal and external events are conditioned cues (triggers) that cause powerful desires (cravings) to use substances.

As a result of changes caused by addiction, common everyday events can trigger memories of the euphoria released by mood-altering brain chemicals. The "good" feeling drives a person to use again and again. This is the fundamental nature of the brain disease in addiction.

Tolerance, Dependence, and Withdrawal

If you take a drug for a certain period of time, your body will adapt to it and grow accustomed to its presence. Over time, you might need a higher dose to get the same effect. This natural response of the body to medication is called *tolerance,* and it's not unique to morphine and the opioids.

If your body has become used to a regular dose of a given medication, stopping abruptly may cause what's known as *withdrawal*. Withdrawal is a collection of symptoms (varying from unpleasant to life-threatening, depending on the drug) that are the body's response to being deprived of a substance to which it has become accustomed. If, for example, a woman who has been taking blood pressure medication for some time suddenly stops doing so, her blood pressure could rise dangerously high and she could have a stroke or heart attack because her body has become dependent on the medication. This is an example of why many types of medicine, not just opioids, should not be stopped suddenly.

If withdrawal symptoms occur when a person stops taking a drug, this is called *dependence*. The amount of time needed to cause dependence varies from drug to drug and from person to person. Dependence is not, however, a disease; it simply means that a person will have withdrawal symptoms if he or she stops taking a given drug.

Addiction, as we've noted, is a behavioral disease characterized by obsessive thoughts and compulsive use of a drug, even when it causes harm. Dependence on a drug, although associated with addiction, is much different from addiction itself.

Some medications used for pain pose no risk at all for addiction. These include anti-inflammatory drugs, antidepressants, and antiseizure medications. However, opioid medications, such as morphine and codeine, can be very addictive. But when they are taken for pain as directed by a physician, the risk of addiction *for the average person* seems to be small, although little research exists in this area. This is definitely *not* the case, however, for people in recovery from alcoholism or other substance abuse. These individuals must be extremely careful about using any opioid (see chapter 8).

Environment and Addiction: A Case Study

A 1972 study by Lee Robins demonstrates an aspect of the connection between environment and addiction.[5] The purpose of the study was to discover how many soldiers had used drugs in Vietnam, what they'd used, how many continued to use drugs after they returned to the United States, and whether they had become or remained addicted since their return.

Robins found that their drug use prior to Vietnam was strongly related to drug use in Vietnam. Of men who used opioids, amphetamines, or barbiturates in Vietnam, more than two-thirds had had prior experience with marijuana, almost one-half with amphetamines, about one-fourth with barbiturates, and one-fifth with opioids. For nearly all of them, however, Vietnam was their first experience with heroin; only 7 percent of users in Vietnam had used it prior to their arrival there.

A surprisingly high proportion of the men who reported having been addicted to heroin in Vietnam, Robins discovered, reported no continuation of addiction once they returned home. The rate of addiction fell tenfold after leaving Vietnam.

In a follow-up study in 1974, Robins found even more encouraging news. Researchers estimated that only about 1.3 percent of all Vietnam returnees had been addicted to narcotics at some time since they returned to the United States, and many of that group reported that they were no longer addicted. Their urinalyses at the follow-up interview confirmed a very low rate of current heroin use.

The men who continued to use opioids after their return were disproportionately those with a previous history of drug use before service, those who did not finish high school, those who had been arrested before they entered service, and those who used amphetamines and barbiturates as well as opioids in Vietnam. Also noted was a significant rate of use of the other drugs above, upon returning home, by these self-described narcotic addicts.

Robins concluded, "The results of this study indicate that dependence on narcotics (opioids) is not so permanent as we had once believed, at least among young healthy men whose period of addiction was less than one year. Not only did many of the addicted men stop their drug use without any special treatment at the time they left Vietnam, but many of those who continued have not been re-addicted."

Although we have learned much about addiction, especially in recent years, questions still remain. Heroin is widely considered one of the most addictive drugs a person can use, along with methamphetamine and nicotine. As this study shows, many young men used heroin extensively for some time while in Vietnam, often to numb the pain and horror of war. Given what we understand about addiction, many should have become addicted. But they didn't. What's more, few had problems with addiction later in their lives. While genetics plays a significant role in an individual's risk of developing addiction—research suggests it accounts for more than half of that risk—environmental factors such as exposure to drugs, family views of intoxication, and cultural factors also compose a portion of the risk.

In the population at large, too, many people who use addictive drugs do not become addicted to them, as shown by the chart on page 40. Note than about 32 percent of those who try tobacco become addicted to it; this is higher than the 23 percent of those who experiment with heroin. Cocaine and alcohol follow with rates of 17 and 15 percent. Addiction research has yet to give us definitive answers as to why this is so, but genetic factors likely play a role.

Treatment

Treatment for addiction to alcohol and other drugs is available in both inpatient and outpatient settings. Most people enter treatment reluctantly, however, because they deny that they have a problem. Health or legal problems may prompt treatment. Intervention helps some alcoholics and addicts recognize and accept the need for treatment.

A wide range of treatments are available to help people

Rates of Nonmedical Drug Experimentation and Dependence

Drug of Abuse	Ever Used (%) *	Dependence among Users (%)*
Tobacco	76	32
Alcohol	92	15
Illicit Drugs	51	15
Cannabis	46	9
Cocaine	16	17
Stimulants	15	11
Anxiolytics	13	9
Analgesics	10	8
Psychedelics	11	5
Heroin	2	23
Inhalants	9	4

rounded to nearest whole number

Adapted from J. C. Anthony, L. A. Warner, and R. C. Kessler, "Comparative Epidemiology of Dependence on Tobacco, Alcohol, Controlled Substances, and Inhalants: Basic Findings from the National Comorbidity Survey," *Experimental and Clinical Psychopharmacology* 2 (1994): 244–68. Chart originally titled "Estimated Prevalence among 15- to 54-Year-Olds of Nonmedical Use and Dependence among Users 1990–1992 (NCS)."

caught in the grip of addiction. Treatment is tailored to the individual; it may involve an evaluation, a brief intervention, an outpatient program or counseling, or a residential inpatient stay.

The first step in treatment is to determine whether individuals are truly addicted. If they are, merely cutting back on use is inappropriate and ineffective, and abstinence must be a crucial part of their treatment goal.

For people who aren't addicted to alcohol or other drugs, but who are experiencing the adverse effects of drinking or using or both, the goal of treatment is to reduce chemical-related problems, often through counseling or a brief intervention. An intervention usually involves drug-abuse specialists who can establish a specific treatment plan. Interventions may include goal setting, behavioral modification techniques, use of mutual-help programs, counseling, and follow-up care at a treatment center.

Most residential alcohol and drug treatment programs in the United States provide detoxification, individual and group therapy, participation in Alcoholics Anonymous (AA), educational lectures, family involvement, work assignments, activity therapy, and the services of counselors—many of whom are recovering alcoholics or addicts and other professional staff. A typical residential treatment program usually includes the components listed below.

Detoxification and withdrawal. Treatment may begin with a program of detoxification, usually lasting about four to seven days. Some clients may be given medications to prevent withdrawal symptoms such as delirium tremens or seizures.

Medical assessment and treatment. Common medical problems related to alcoholism and drug addiction are high blood pressure, elevated blood sugar, liver and heart disease, HIV, and hepatitis C.

Psychological support and psychiatric treatment. Group and individual counseling and therapy support a person's recovery from the psychological aspects of addiction. Emotional symptoms of the disease may mimic psychiatric disorders, and some people may have a specific psychiatric illness in addition to their addiction.

Emphasis on acceptance and abstinence. Effective treatment is impossible unless people understand that they're addicted and unable to control their substance use and that they must totally abstain from using alcohol or any other drug. In fact, abstinence is the stated goal of most addiction treatment programs, but for people with chronic pain, an exception may need to be made in relation to the use of prescription medication.

Drug treatments. An alcohol-sensitizing drug called disulfiram (Antabuse) may be a strong deterrent. Disulfiram will neither cure alcoholism nor remove the compulsion to drink. But in those who drink alcohol, the drug produces a severe physical reaction that includes flushing, nausea, vomiting, and headaches. Naltrexone (ReVia), a drug long known to block the action of morphine and the opioids, also reduces a recovering alcoholic's urge to drink. Unlike disulfiram, naltrexone doesn't make people feel sick soon after taking a drink. Naltrexone is also used in recovery from narcotic addiction because it blocks the high from opioids. It's also important to note that when patients on naltrexone take opioid medications for pain, they may not experience pain relief. In fact, when people who use opioids regularly take naltrexone, they could experience sudden, extreme withdrawal.

Continuing support. Aftercare programs and AA help recovering alcoholics and addicts abstain from alcohol and other drugs, manage relapses, and cope with necessary lifestyle changes. The more we learn about addiction treatment, the more we realize it must be long lasting. Addiction is a chronic illness requiring long-term care to ensure ongoing abstinence and continued improvement in psychosocial functioning.

Recovery: A Lifelong Journey

Recovery comes in stages, one step at a time. Each new level brings new challenges to address. In the early stages of recovery, it's not unusual for people to find that life seems dull and discouraging. In time, however, and with effort, life can become more rich and rewarding than they ever expected.

During the more difficult times, many people see only the challenges of the moment. It seems all too easy to fall back into old ways and habits. That's when courage, self-discipline, and help from others have to carry them through. People need to learn to mentally record and cherish the new energy that they feel when moving ahead. To help them through the tough times, they can relive the pride and happiness they've felt by staying off alcohol and other drugs, and they can look back at how far they've come.

During recovery, addicts may believe that their problem is merely with their particular drug of choice. An alcoholic, for example, might stop drinking and think that using a different drug, such as marijuana, will be fine. We now know, however, that addiction is *independent* of the substance abused. Changing to a different drug is no solution; the addict will simply continue the addictive behavior with the new drug. In order to overcome addictive behavior, people must leave behind more than their particular addiction or drug of choice. They must give up all addictive drugs along with their addictive behaviors.

Recovery is more than abstinence. That's just the first step on the road to a better life. Without deeper changes in their lives, people may stop addictive behaviors, but they won't be able to "stay stopped" with comfort. Recovery requires that people both stop their addictive behavior *and* deal with the needs that their addiction was supposed to fulfill. Without meeting these challenges, all the issues that they carried around but did not face will remain unresolved.

Making such a profound change is not like simply flipping a light switch: "Yesterday I was an addict, but now I'm not. I'm done with that." Overcoming addiction and living in recovery is a lifelong process that requires persistent attention and effort.

Relapse

Relapse is the process of returning to the use of alcohol or other drugs after having quit for a time. Relapse warning signs may involve a person's behavior, attitudes, feelings, or thoughts, or a combination of all of them. When these warning signs arise, it doesn't necessarily mean that a person is going to relapse, but he or she needs to pay attention and do something about them to prevent a relapse. Many alcoholics and drug addicts who have relapsed know that there were many clues to relapse long before it happened. Relapse is always possible, no matter how long a person has been sober.

Finding Support

Recovery is a *process,* and there are points in that process where outside help is necessary. Many recovering alcoholics and their family members find that participating in support groups is an essential part of coping with the disease, preventing or dealing with relapse, and staying sober.

Alcoholics Anonymous

The fellowship of Alcoholics Anonymous (AA) was formed in 1935. As a mutual help group of recovering alcoholics, AA offers a sober peer group as an effective model for achieving total abstinence: "Alcoholics Anonymous is a fellowship of men and women who share their experience, strength, and hope with one another in order to solve their common problem and to help others to recover from alcoholism. The only requirement for membership is a desire to stop drinking. There are no dues or fees for AA membership; it is self-supporting through its own contributions. AA is not allied with any sect, denomination, politics, organization, or institution. [Members'] primary purpose is to stay sober and help other alcoholics to achieve sobriety."[6]

The AA program is built around the Twelve Steps, straight-forward suggestions for men and women who choose to lead sober lives (see appendix F). Following the Twelve Steps of AA isn't required for membership; rather, they are *suggested steps* for people who choose to live sober lives. As guides to recovery, the Steps help alcoholics accept their powerlessness over alcohol. They stress the necessity for honesty about the past and present.

AA is not a religion; it is, however, a deeply spiritual program that offers a way of life rather than the path of formal religion, and as such, it continues to be embraced by representatives of many different denominations. The Twelve Steps include principles of humility, self-examination, restitution, and living the spiritual principle that people ultimately cannot help themselves except by helping others. Recovery in AA is based on accepting the unique experience of each alcoholic. Through listening to and sharing stories, alcoholics learn that they aren't alone.

Family members of recovering alcoholics have formed a complementary mutual help group called Al-Anon. Al-Anon is designed for people who are affected by someone else's alcoholism. In sharing their stories, they gain a greater understanding of how the disease affects the entire family, not just the alcoholic. Al-Anon also accepts the Twelve Steps as the principles by which participants are to conduct their lives. It emphasizes the need to learn detachment and forgiveness if people are to be free of the disease. In many communities, Alateen groups are also available, geared to teenage children of alcoholics.

Over the years, many support groups based on the AA philosophy and the Twelve Steps have formed to help people recover from other addictions. They include Cocaine Anonymous, Narcotics Anonymous, Overeaters Anonymous, Gamblers Anonymous, and Debtors Anonymous. Doctors or counselors can refer patients to such support groups. These groups are also commonly listed in the phone book, in the local newspaper, and on the Web.

Narcotics Anonymous

Narcotics Anonymous (NA) is an international, community-based association of recovering drug addicts with more than 31,000 weekly meetings in more than one hundred countries worldwide. It sprang from the Alcoholics Anonymous program of the late 1940s, with meetings first emerging in the Los Angeles area in the early 1950s.

Membership is open to all drug addicts, regardless of the particular drug or combination of drugs used. When adapting AA's First Step, the word *addiction* was substituted for *alcohol*, thus removing drug-specific language and reflecting the disease concept of addiction.

As with AA, NA has no social, religious, economic, racial, ethnic, national, gender, or class status membership restrictions. There are no dues or fees for membership. While most members regularly contribute small sums to help cover the expenses of meetings, such contributions are not mandatory.

The NA recovery process is inextricably linked to a support network. One of the keys to NA's success is the therapeutic value of addicts working with other addicts. Members share their successes and challenges in overcoming active addiction and living drug-free, productive lives through the application of the principles contained within the Twelve Steps of NA.

Principles incorporated within the Steps include

- admitting there is a problem
- seeking help
- engaging in a thorough self-examination
- particiating in confidential self-disclosure
- making amends for harm done
- helping other drug addicts who want to recover

Central to the NA program is its emphasis on practicing spiritual principles. NA itself is nonreligious, but each member is encouraged to cultivate an individual understanding, religious or not, of this "spiritual awakening."

NA is not affiliated with other organizations, including other Twelve Step programs, treatment centers, or correctional facilities. As an organization, NA neither employs professional counselors or therapists nor provides residential facilities or clinics. Additionally, the fellowship does not provide vocational, legal, financial, psychiatric, or medical services. NA has only one mission: provide an environment in which addicts can help one another to stop using drugs and find a new way to live.

NA members are encouraged to comply with complete abstinence from all drugs, including alcohol. It has been the experience of NA members that complete and continuous abstinence provides the best foundation for recovery and personal growth. As a whole, NA takes no position on outside issues, including prescribed medications. Use of psychiatric medication and other medically indicated drugs prescribed by a physician and taken under medical supervision is not seen as compromising a person's recovery in NA.[7]

Those in recovery from addiction to alcohol and/or other drugs already understand the power of these substances. A recovering person coping with acute or chronic pain may have serious concerns about any medication that could trigger a relapse . . . and with good reason! In the next chapter, we will begin discussing pain medications, and in chapter 5, we will explore ways to treat pain with complementary medicine techniques. As you will see, there are many ways to address pain without resorting to medications that are potentially addictive or that could trigger a relapse for someone in recovery.

CHAPTER 4

Pain Medications

Carlos, whose drugs of choice were alcohol and cocaine, has been sober for nearly fifteen years. As part of his recovery program, he has tried to avoid all drugs or medications. At forty-five, he's had the good fortune to have few medical problems during his life. About a year ago, however, he sprained his wrist playing volleyball. The injury didn't heal as he hoped, and he was frustrated by ongoing and occasionally severe pain in the joint. Carlos put off doing anything at all about the pain. He was simply "gutting it out" until one day, a friend who worked for a drug treatment center suggested he take ibuprofen. The next day, Carlos called his friend and exclaimed, "My God, does that stuff work great! It completely relieved the pain I've had for weeks now. It's just gone."

Over-the-counter (nonprescription) pain medications *are* effective, and Carlos simply had no idea how helpful this class of drugs can be. He's not alone. Many people, especially people in recovery, who often have a healthy reluctance to turn to any drugs for pain relief, don't realize that researchers have made remarkable advances in pain relief medication. Many effective nonaddictive medications are available today to relieve pain.

Yes, times have changed! In recent years, our understanding of pain has grown immensely. Today, we have a broad array of effective options for treating chronic pain. One of these, of course, is medication. When used appropriately, medications can help people reduce their pain with limited side effects. They can also help people control temporary recurrences of pain and treat other problems that accompany chronic pain, such as insomnia and depression.

For acute pain, medication is often the first treatment choice. For chronic pain, medications might serve as part of a broader treatment package including exercise, physical therapy, behavior changes, and other nonpharmacological physical treatments. Although medications can be helpful, they aren't cure-alls, they can cause side effects, and they may be costly.

In this chapter, you'll find information on specific medications, including

- simple analgesics
- topical medications
- "adjuvant" medications that help pain treatment
- medications for other pain-related symptoms
- opioids

We will begin by discussing drugs that have little or no potential for triggering relapse or causing addiction. Then we will consider those with the greatest potential for harm—the opioids—and their possible usefulness as part of a broad treatment plan.

Indeed, it is important to regard drugs of any kind as part of a broader plan for pain control, particularly when pain is chronic. Work with your doctor and other medical providers to develop a plan that uses all the tools available to you, including rehabilitative therapies, complementary or alternative medicine (CAM), and psychological and cognitive behavioral therapies.

Today, it is common for people to use CAM in conjunction with the pain-relief care they receive from their doctor; some use CAM exclusively. (See chapter 5 for more information on this field of medicine.)

Psychological or cognitive behavioral therapies that address pain are designed principally to improve function, regardless of pain. This behavioristic approach may involve learning coping and stress-reduction techniques and examining attitudes about your overall life situation. Even if the pain can't be eliminated, there are still a number of changes you can make in your attitude toward your circumstances and in your behavior that can greatly improve your life. (See chapter 6 for more information on this topic.)

Simple Analgesics

The term *analgesic* means "pain-reliever." Simple, nonopioid analgesics offer a good starting point when looking at pain medications. They are usually the first ones recommended for people who have pain, and they are not addictive. They include acetaminophen and anti-inflammatory medications such as aspirin. Another term for aspirin and its relatives is *nonsteroidal anti-inflammatory drugs* (NSAIDs).

NSAIDs

NSAIDs reduce inflammation and relieve pain and fever. They are most effective for mild to moderate pain accompanied by swelling and inflammation. These drugs work by inhibiting an enzyme called *cyclooxygenase (COX)*. This enzyme is responsible for producing *prostaglandins,* hormonelike substances involved in inflammation and pain. Many drugs in this class require a prescription, but some NSAIDs are available over the counter. NSAIDs are especially helpful for arthritis and pain resulting from muscle sprains, strains, back and neck injuries, or cramps.

Over-the-counter NSAIDs include the following:

- aspirin
- ibuprofen (Advil, Motrin, and others)
- ketoprofen (Orudis)
- naproxen sodium (Aleve)

NSAIDs available only by prescription include the following:

- diclofenac potassium (Cataflam)
- diclofenac sodium (Voltaren)
- etodolac (Lodine)
- flurbiprofen (Ansaid)
- indomethacin (Indocin)
- ketorolac (Toradol, Acular)
- nabumetone (Relafen)
- naproxen (Anaprox, Naprelan, Naprosyn)
- oxaprozin (Daypro)
- piroxicam (Feldene)
- sulindac (Clinoril)

When taken as directed, NSAIDs are generally safe. But if you exceed the recommended dosage—and sometimes even if you adhere to the recommended dosage—NSAIDs can cause nausea, stomach pain, stomach bleeding, or ulcers. Large doses can lead to kidney problems and fluid retention, and this risk increases with age. If you regularly take NSAIDs, talk to your doctor so that you can be monitored for side effects.

NSAIDs have a "ceiling effect," a limit to how much pain they can control. This means that beyond a certain dosage, they don't provide additional benefit. If you have moderate to severe pain, exceeding the dosage limit may not help relieve your pain. In chapter 1, we looked at how inflammation can sensitize nociceptors and increase pain. By blocking inflammation, we often create a pain-relieving effect. Aspirin and other NSAIDs will block both pain and inflammation and will also reduce fever. All NSAIDs share these properties.

Common NSAID Side Effects

Platelets are the cells in the blood that are necessary for clotting. Platelet function depends on prostaglandins and therefore NSAIDs have an antiplatelet effect; they impair blood clotting. This can be beneficial, particularly for patients with heart disease. Your doctor might have you take an aspirin a day to prevent heart attacks.

Taken excessively, however, NSAIDs can cause bleeding problems in two ways—not only because of the antiplatelet effect, but also because most NSAIDs block prostaglandin E, a normal chemical in the stomach that protects the stomach lining from digestive acids. NSAIDs, therefore, can increase the risk of ulcers.

NSAIDs can be taken with food or milk to reduce the risk of gastrointestinal side effects. Your doctor may prescribe medication to decrease acid secretion in the stomach, for example, lansoprazole (Prevacid) or omeprazole (Prilosec). A doctor may also suggest taking a medication that includes prostaglandin E or misoprostol to decrease gastrointestinal side effects. Unfortunately, these medications can also cause diarrhea and cramping.

Because of the anti-clotting effects of NSAIDs, people who take them may notice that they bleed or bruise more easily. Large doses of NSAIDs can also lead to kidney problems and fluid retention, which can worsen congestive heart failure. NSAIDs can cause liver function abnormalities, as well as ringing in the ears, headache, dizziness, and drowsiness. Mouth sores and skin rashes also can occur while taking NSAIDs.

Acetaminophen

Acetaminophen—which goes by the trade name Tylenol, among others—is often grouped with anti-inflammatory drugs, but it does not reduce inflammation. Rather, it is a pain reliever that also reduces fever. Acetaminophen is most effective for mild to moderate pain that isn't accompanied by inflammation.

When taken occasionally and as recommended, acetaminophen is quite safe. It does not affect platelets or blood clotting. Acetaminophen is nonaddictive, doesn't cause drowsiness, is usually very well tolerated, doesn't harm the stomach, and is an excellent frontline pain reliever. However, people who frequently take more of the drug than recommended (4,000 mg per day) risk liver damage. In fact, in high doses, it can do irreversible harm to the liver, and an overdose of acetaminophen can be lethal. Taking acetaminophen with alcohol increases the risk of liver damage and can lead to liver failure.

A variety of over-the-counter and prescription medications may contain acetaminophen, including cold remedies, pain relievers, and sleeping aids. It's therefore important to calculate a total daily use of acetaminophen from all sources. Read the ingredient label of all medications you take.

Both acetaminophen and NSAIDs are quite effective in moderate doses. While safe for recovering addicts or alcoholics, either one, taken inappropriately and/or in high doses, can be very harmful.

COX-2 Inhibitors

Newer versions of NSAIDs called COX-2 inhibitors became available a few years ago. Researchers discovered that cyclooxygenase comes in two forms: COX-1 and COX-2. Part of the role of COX-1 is to protect the stomach lining and enable platelet function. Because the other NSAIDs suppress its function, side effects such as stomach problems and lower blood-clotting rates can result from NSAIDs. But COX-2 inhibitors affect only the form of the enzyme involved in pain and inflammation. Because they don't affect COX-1, COX-2 inhibitors may lower the risk of gastrointestinal and other bleeding problems. However, the COX-2 inhibitors may create a higher risk of cardiovascular complications such as heart attack or stroke, especially if they are used for a prolonged time. The only COX-2 inhibitor currently on the market is celecoxib (Celebrex).

Topical Medications

Topical medications are creams or gels that can be applied directly to the skin. These drugs act on the surface of the body and work within the skin. Topical pain-relief ointments can occasionally help relieve nerve pain and inflammation located just below the surface of the skin. They are all nonaddictive and generally safe. Three types of topical medications are available: local anesthetics, topical analgesics, and counter-irritant products.

Local Anesthetics

Local anesthetics block the electrical conduction of nerve signals.

Lidocaine patches (such as Lidoderm) are commonly prescribed for relief of pain associated with neuralgia and nerve pain.

EMLA is a prescription pain-relief cream made from two topical anesthetics: lidocaine and prilocaine. Usually within an hour after it's applied, the skin becomes numb. The benefits are greatest two to three hours after application. EMLA is commonly used to reduce pain before giving an injection, drawing blood, inserting an intravenous line, or treating a wart.

Over-the-counter products that are available for pain relief include dibucaine (Nupercainal), lidocaine (Xylocaine, Zilactin-L), benzocaine (Lanacane, Solarcaine), and pramoxine (Prax, Itch-X).

Topical Analgesics

Trolamine salicylate, a chemical similar to aspirin, is the active ingredient in such medications as Aspercreme, Sportscreme, and Myoflex. The Food and Drug Administration (FDA) lists these drugs as safe but not necessarily effective for pain relief. They are available over the counter.

Counterirritant Products

These nonprescription medications, such as ArthriCare, BenGay, and Icy Hot, stimulate the receptors in the body that sense heat or cold in order to cover up or counteract pain. Counterirritant products may relieve occasional, mild muscle aches, but they're not effective for most forms of chronic pain. In addition, they typically require frequent applications.[1]

Capsaicin (Zostrix), a nonprescription drug, is made from the seeds of hot chili peppers. It's thought to work by depleting the body's nerve cells of a chemical called substance P, which has a role in transmitting pain messages. Capsaicin is most effective for temporary relief of arthritic pain in joints close to the skin's surface, such as the fingers, knees, and elbows. Some people report that capsaicin helps relieve pain after shingles (postherpetic neuralgia), pain from diabetes (diabetic neuropathy), and chronic pain near healed surgical scars.

Adjuvant Medications

Interestingly, some of the more effective and commonly used medications for chronic pain are drugs that were developed to treat other conditions. Among these are antidepressants. In addition to relieving symptoms of depression, these drugs have been found to interfere with certain chemical processes in your brain and spinal cord that affect how you feel pain.

Tricyclic antidepressants relieve pain at dosages that are too low to have an effect on depression. In fact, newer medications called SSRIs—selective serotonin reuptake inhibitors— have far fewer side effects than do tricyclic antidepressants.

While the SSRI antidepressants work best for depression, they do not work very well for pain.

The tricyclic antidepressants most commonly used for pain management are amitriptyline (Amitril, Elavil) and nortriptyline (Aventyl, Pamelor). Others used on occasion for treating chronic pain include the following:

- desipramine (Pertofrane, Norpramin)
- doxepin (Sinequan, Adapin)
- imipramine (Janamine, Tofranil)
- protriptyline (Vivactil)
- trimipramine (Surmontil)
- clomipramine (Anafranil)

Antidepressants don't cause dependence or addiction. However, tricyclic antidepressants can cause drowsiness. Therefore, it's generally recommended that patients take the medication in the evening before bed. In addition, these drugs may cause dry mouth, constipation, weight gain, difficulty with urination, and changes in blood pressure. Side effects usually begin soon after starting the medication or when a dose is increased, but pain relief may not occur for several weeks.

To reduce or prevent side effects, your doctor will likely start at a low dose and slowly increase the amount. Most people are able to take tricyclic antidepressants, particularly in low doses, with only mild side effects.

Antiseizure Medications

Antiseizure (anticonvulsant) medications were developed primarily to reduce or control epileptic seizures, but they also help control stabbing or burning pain from nerve damage. These drugs seem to work by quieting damaged nerves to slow or prevent uncontrolled pain signals.

Antiseizure medications used for chronic pain include the following:

- carbamazepine (Carbatrol, Tegretol)
- divalproex sodium (Depakote)
- gabapentin (Neurontin)
- lamotrigine (Lamictal)
- phenytoin (Dilantin)
- oxcarbazepine (Trileptal)
- tiagabine (Gabitril)
- topiramate (Topamax)
- valproic acid (Depakene)

These drugs also have another major advantage: they are quite safe. They sometimes cause a bit of dizziness or drowsiness, nausea, or impaired balance and coordination, but they are generally well tolerated. Most people are bothered only minimally. More severe but less common side effects include blood and liver disorders.

Generally speaking, this is a large class of many different drugs. Some are safer than others, some more effective than others, but all have the advantage of not being subject to abuse.

Opioids: Some Distinctions

Before addressing the complex topic of opioid pain medications, it's important to clarify our terminology. What are the differences between opioids, opiates, opium, and narcotics?

Opium is a natural plant compound derived from the opium poppy.[2] Derivatives of the poppy, first cultivated around 3400 BCE, have been used by humans for thousands of years. The word *opium* is derived from the Greek word meaning "juice of a plant." Ancient Sumerians, Assyrians, Babylonians, and Egyptians learned that smoking opium caused pleasurable effects. Use of the plant later spread to Arabia, India, and China. In Europe, it was reintroduced by Paracelsus (1493–1541). In the 1700s, opium smoking was popular in parts of Asia, and the opium trade was an important source of income for colonial rulers from England, Holland, and Spain.

Opium contains a considerable number of substances, which were finally isolated in the 1800s. Friedrich Sertürner was the first to extract one of these substances in a pure form. He called this chemical morphine, after Morpheus, the Greek god of sleep or dreams. Morphine is the active pain-relieving substance in opium. Drugs derived from opium are called *opiates*. Scientists have also created synthetic compounds that structurally resemble morphine and work in similar ways but don't come from a plant at all. *Opioids,* the preferred term for these compounds, include both the natural and synthetic forms.

People soon realized that morphine was addictive and began looking for a nonaddictive opiate by altering morphine's structure. In 1874, an English pharmacist, C. R. Alder Wright, boiled morphine and acetic acid to produce diacetylmorphine. This new compound was soon manufactured and marketed under the brand name Heroin. Heroin was initially sold as a cough suppressant and quickly became popular. It was sold worldwide until it became obvious that people were overusing it. The Bayer pharmaceutical company stopped distribution in 1913.

Thus we have opium, the natural plant extract; opiates, which are compounds purified from the plant, such as morphine; and opioids, which include drugs that are structurally related but don't actually derive from the plant; instead they may be synthesized in the laboratory.

All of these compounds, which historically were called narcotics, have properties of reducing pain and inducing sleepiness. The term *narcotic* is still technically correct. However, it is no longer used in the addiction field, first because it has acquired negative connotations associated with illegal drug use. Second, the U.S. Drug Enforcement Administration includes not only morphine and its relatives in that category, but also cocaine, LSD, and marijuana, which are not related to the opioids. Therefore, we will refer to morphine and its relatives as opioids rather than narcotics.

The human body contains naturally occurring chemicals called opioid peptides, which are similar to morphine. These peptides, the endorphins and enkephalins, bind to the same receptors as morphine in the brain and spinal cord, blocking pain pathways.

The Weak Opioids

As we move up in the level of medication strength, we enter the opioid world. The weak opioids, such as codeine and propoxyphene (Darvocet), are medications often prescribed by family practitioners and internists for acute pain. These weak opioids are effective for pain, but they are usually used only for short-term pain problems. People with a history of alcohol or other drug abuse need to be careful when taking weak opioids. These medications represent a cautionary zone.

Tramadol (Ultram) is a prescription pain medication that works in two ways. Like a weak opioid, it interferes with the transmission of pain signals. The drug also increases levels of norepinephrine and serotonin neurotransmitters that help reduce pain like a tricyclic antidepressant. Tramadol is used mainly to relieve mild to moderate pain. The risk of physical dependence and addiction with tramodol is less than with opioids, but it is nevertheless possible. Side effects from tramadol can include dizziness, sedation, headache, nausea, constipation, and seizures. Possible long-term effects from the drug are unknown.

The weak opioids, however, work at the same opioid receptors as morphine. Unlike the previous categories of pain-relieving medications, there is potential for abuse. Because the weak opioids are just that—weak—they may seem less risky than strong opioids like morphine. With the latter, you know you're dealing with a powerful drug. It's tempting, however, to use the weak opioids carelessly rather than exactly as prescribed by your doctor. It's easy to think that because they're routinely prescribed, they won't cause any problem.

Bill, a forty-two-year-old accountant, went to see an orthopedist for a jammed thumb and some knee pain after a Saturday of playing touch football with friends. He told the doctor about his alcoholic past. Upon hearing this background, his doctor said, "Well, I'm very glad you told me, because normally I prescribe acetaminophen (Tylenol) with codeine for a problem like yours, but given your history, I don't want to do that." He asked Bill to use only ibuprofen instead and see if it would give him adequate pain relief. Bill was relieved, saying that he didn't think he needed something as strong as Tylenol with codeine, and that he was nervous about taking any opioid.

Acetaminophen with codeine might have given Bill somewhat faster and better pain relief, but only with significant risk to his sobriety. Even with commonly prescribed weak opioids, it's important to have an honest, open discussion with your doctor. He or she needs to know about any past drug abuse, even if it was "only" with alcohol. A low dose of a weak opioid can still trigger relapse, whether or not you ever used opioids. Because these drugs are prescribed more freely than the strong opioids, it's even more important that your doctor know about any addiction background.

The Moderate Opioids

The moderate opioids are more potent and are often combined with acetaminophen. By combining the drug with acetaminophen, the potential for intravenous drug abuse is lowered. That is why oxycodone with acetaminophen (Percocet) is in the moderate class, but pure oxycodone (OxyContin) is considered a strong opioid.

Acetaminophen is sometimes combined with an opioid to provide stronger pain relief. These drugs are available only by prescription. Whenever you use a combination of medications, ask your doctor and pharmacist about the use and side effects of each. For example, make sure you're not taking too much acetaminophen.

Moderate opioids include the following:

- oxycodone with acetaminophen (Percocet)
- hydrocodone with acetaminophen (Vicodin)

The Strong Opioids

The strong opioids have no ceiling, meaning that they can relieve pain as intense as it comes. Strong opioids are often used to relieve pain from cancer, terminal illness, severe injury, or surgery. Pain control after surgery is especially important because it allows you to be active more quickly, and the sooner you're active, the less you're at risk for complications, such as pneumonia or blood clots, due to inactivity.

Frequently prescribed strong opioids include the following:

- fentanyl (Duragesic)
- hydromorphone (Dilaudid)
- meperidine (Demerol)
- methadone (Dolophine)
- morphine (MS Contin, Oramorph SR, MSIR)
- oxycodone (OxyContin, OxyIR)
- oxymorphone (Numorphan)

Factors Important in Choosing the Best Opioid

Determining Length of Effectiveness

The duration of a medicine's action is an important factor because it determines how often a patient will have to take it. Many medicines come in immediate-release and sustained-delivery formulations. Morphine, for example, in MS Contin form, provides a slow release over about eight hours. The immediate-release form, MSIR, on the other hand, is absorbed quickly but lasts for only two or three hours. OxyContin provides sustained release of oxycodone for twelve hours, and OxyIR is an immediate-release formulation that lasts three to four hours.

In general, slow-release, infrequently dosed formulations are preferred for chronic pain because they are more convenient and may have less likelihood of abuse. Slow-release formulations reduce the behavioral connection between feeling pain, taking a pill, and getting a quick response (pain relief). Many physicians prefer drugs such as methadone, OxyContin, MS Contin, and the fentanyl patch because they provide a long duration of action without creating rapid changes in the level of the drug in the patient's body. This may also minimize side effects.

Of course, slow-release medications like OxyContin can still be abused when a patient intentionally crushes the drug and either inhales it through the nose or takes more than the recommended amount. Because the continuous-release forms have to contain enough drug to last for an extended period of time, the absolute amount of drug in a given dose is higher. It's just trickled out slowly over time. So if you try to get it all at once, you can actually have a higher risk of overdose or addiction than with the immediate-release formulations.

Addressing Breakthrough Pain

Some people may experience *breakthrough pain,* which rises abruptly above a person's baseline pain level. Most often, people with breakthrough pain are already using a sustained-release medicine formulation that is effective most of the time.

When pain "breaks through" that medication, patients may be instructed to take additional quick-acting/short-duration medication.

This situation increases risk for two reasons. First, short-acting medications enter the brain more quickly, and so have the potential to be more addicting. Second, taking medications in response to pain strengthens the behavioral connection to the reward pathways.

Ideally, then, you would want to choose a nonpharmacological option to treat breakthrough pain. Alternatively, a nonopioid medication would be a better choice than opioids in such a situation. Ask your doctor whether breakthrough pain is a possibility. If it is, this situation must be fully discussed. It's very important to create specific guidelines for the use of breakthrough pain medication. If shorter-acting opioids are used, your supply of medicine should be limited. You might be given only ten tablets, for example. Your support people—spouse, friends, family members—should be involved and understand the situation, too. You should have very clear limits on dosage and frequency. If you find yourself wanting to go beyond these guidelines, you need to call your doctor.

Important Information about Meperidine (Demerol) and Methadone

Meperidine (Demerol) is metabolized to a toxic derivative product called normeperidine that can cause seizures. People considering taking meperidine should do so only under the close care of a doctor. People with impaired kidney function or a history of seizures should not take meperidine.

As a strong opioid, methadone is an excellent medication for chronic pain because it has a long duration of action in the body and it's inexpensive. Unfortunately, it's commonly associated with heroin addiction programs and therefore has some negative connotations. Nevertheless, methadone is a legitimate and *very* effective pain medication. In addition, it has a particular advantage for chronic pain management because it provides some relief for neuropathic pain as well as somatic pain. Furthermore, it seems to be less likely to cause tolerance than other opioids.

Route of Delivery

Physicians have a number of choices for administering pain medications, from injection with needles to sophisticated devices such as infusion pumps. Each has its advantages.

Oral Medications

Oral delivery of medication is the most preferable method, primarily because it's inexpensive, simple, and easy to understand. When a drug is taken orally, it goes through the stomach and the intestines, where part of it is metabolized before it even reaches the nervous system. Once the medication is in the bloodstream, only a tiny fraction will pass through the blood-brain barrier to the brain and spinal cord. Because the intestines are thus heavily exposed to the drug, constipation can be a significant problem.

For patients who have intolerable intestinal side effects or who can't take medicine orally, doctors can change to a delivery route that doesn't use the intestines. Certain opioids can be inhaled, such as pentazocine (Talwin) and buprenorphine

(Buprenex) nasal sprays. Also available are transdermal delivery devices such as the fentanyl patch (Duragesic). There are transmucosal formulations like the fentanyl oralette (Actiq, also called the fentanyl lollipop), and suppository forms of some medications are also available.

Injections

When doctors and other medical providers talk about injections, they are usually specifying a route of delivery—into a muscle (intramuscular), into a vein (intravenous), or just under the skin (subcutaneous), for example, as opposed to taking a medication by mouth, in pill form or as a liquid. These routes are usually used for hospitalized patients when the oral route is unavailable, such as after surgery.

When treating pain, doctors sometimes choose injections to deliver a completely different class of drugs that reduce inflammation: corticosteroids, which are potent anti-inflammatory agents. The COX inhibitors are called nonsteroidal anti-inflammatory drugs (NSAIDs) to distinguish them from steroids like cortisone. An injection of cortisone provides the most potent anti-inflammatory effect possible. It is nearly always given by injection in the area where the inflammation is occurring. Steroids' serious systemic side effects can be minimized when they are injected near the site of the problem, such as near a damaged spinal disk or into an irritated muscle or a joint.

Injections can be effective for intense pain for a short period of time, but they don't usually control pain in the long run. They are most effective for joint, muscle, or nerve pain or for inflammation that's confined to a specific location. One important benefit of injections is that the medicine works mainly in a limited part of the body. By affecting only a specific area rather than the whole body, injections can reduce the amount of medication needed, as well as the number and intensity of side effects.

Spinal Infusion Devices

With a spinal infusion device, morphine or one of its relatives can be placed directly into the spinal fluid. This technique has the advantage of allowing therapeutic concentrations of a drug to be delivered right to the point where it will work in the spinal cord without exposing the rest of the body to very high levels, thus minimizing some side effects. Most often, these devices are placed surgically in the lower abdomen. They can be programmed to provide an adjustable flow of medication, typically an opioid, to the spinal column.

Adverse Effects of Opioids

Side effects of opioids include constipation, itching, nausea, dizziness, drowsiness, sedation, and unclear thinking. While your doctor is adjusting the dose, it's not safe to drive, use heavy equipment, or make any important decisions until you realize how the medication may be affecting you.

All opioids have the potential for abuse and addiction. Heroin and oxycodone are very similar in their risk for addiction. Methadone and buprenorphine, which are used to treat opioid addiction, are less likely to be abused.

Tolerance, Dependence, and Addiction

Three terms relevant to discussion of opioid use are often confused: *tolerance, dependence,* and *addiction* (these terms were noted in chapter 3). Though sometimes inappropriately used synonymously, they actually describe three different conditions.

Tolerance develops when the initial dose of a drug loses its effectiveness over time. As a result, higher doses of the drug are needed to produce the desired effect.

Dependence occurs when a person's body adapts to the long-term presence of a drug. When the drug is withdrawn, he or she can then experience anxiety, headaches, nervousness, shakiness, and other physical withdrawal symptoms. The headaches that a heavy coffee drinker experiences after giving up coffee are a mild sign of physical dependence.

Addiction is a disease marked by cravings for a drug and compulsive use of that drug despite repeated, harmful consequences.

With time, people who take opioids are likely to develop tolerance and even dependence. However, this does *not* mean that they are addicted. Addiction results from many factors— genetic, psychological, and environmental. Exposure to opioids is only one factor. The vast majority of people treated with opioids for pain never become addicted.

Sometimes people with chronic pain act in ways that are mistaken for addiction. These individuals may focus on maintaining their supply of opioids or closely watch the clock in anticipation of their next dose of medication. Generally, however, even these actions are not addictive behaviors but rather are called "pseudoaddiction," because the behaviors stop once people get satisfactory pain relief. (See chapter 8 for more information on pseudoaddiction.)

Opioids and Relapse

Can opioids trigger relapse in people who've abused alcohol only? In short, yes! In some ways, opioids are more of a risk than alcohol, because often recovering alcoholics don't consider "drugs" a risk. Too many alcoholics still mistakenly believe that they won't have a problem with opioids because they never abused them, but that's not the case.

Our current understanding of addiction suggests that all these addictive drugs work through the same part of the brain. Even though alcohol affects different brain receptors than opioids do, these two systems are closely linked since they affect the reward center of the brain.

Researchers today believe that no matter which drug (or drugs) a person is addicted to, the addictive process itself can be triggered by alcohol or any other drug, even one different from what had been a person's "drug of choice." An alcoholic who had never touched any other drugs might, for example, have surgery or need pain medication for dental work. He could have an opioid prescribed for postoperative pain, only to discover that he "loves" the medication. Before he knows it, he is addicted to it. We will discuss the risks of opioids in more detail in chapter 8.

Nerve Stimulators

Nerve stimulators include transcutaneous electronic nerve stimulators (TENS), peripheral nerve stimulators, and spinal cord stimulators. While not affecting all types of pain, these tools have the advantage of controlling pain without the use of drugs. Stimulating nerves and/or the spinal cord can manipulate the "gate" and thereby modulate pain signals. Certain patterns and frequencies of stimulation can mask or "drown out" pain signals. Other theories suggest that electrical stimulation may prompt release of the body's endogenous opioid system.

For nerve stimulation with TENS units, electrodes are placed on the skin near the painful area. A small, battery-powered unit creates painless electrical impulses that pass through the skin to nearby nerve pathways.

Peripheral nerve stimulators work like TENS, but the electrodes are implanted surgically near a peripheral nerve. Spinal cord stimulation involves putting the electrode in the epidural space, which is in the vertebral column.

The technologies discussed in this chapter for treating pain don't necessarily exclude one another. For instance, someone with chronic pain could use a TENS unit together with a pain medication. A decision about what's best should be reached after a conversation between patient and doctor that explores a number of factors, including

- patient expectations
- a medical evaluation
- medical risks and side effects
- the patient's range of pain
- the patient's comfort level
- insurance coverage

Other Factors to Consider When Choosing Pain Medication

When prescribing medications for pain, doctors have to keep in mind a number of factors. Understanding them can help you work better with your doctor to treat your pain.

Rehabilitation and functional recovery. Treatment for chronic pain should not be designed solely to suppress your symptoms. Rather, the greater goal is to help you lead as full and active a life as possible. Pain medication can help you return to your full work schedule, maintain your relationships, and manage the tasks of daily living.

Interactions with other medicines. Doctors and pharmacists always try to avoid drug combinations that cause unsafe interactions, unwanted effects that can occur when some drugs are taken together. For example, many medications include acetaminophen. Make sure you aren't taking too much. Most people should take less than 4,000 mg per day; those with liver problems should take still less. Interactions with over-the-counter medicines, alcohol, and certain foods can also cause problems, so be sure to talk with your doctor or pharmacist about potential problems. Tell your doctor about all the medicines you're taking, including nonprescription drugs and/or supplements.

Allergies. If you are allergic to a medication, obviously you should not take it. But not all adverse reactions are allergic. For example, if ibuprofen causes stomach upset, this is not an allergy. Similarly, nausea or vomiting is not a sign of allergy to opioids—rather, it is a side effect. Having side effects with one member of a class of drugs does not mean you will necessarily have side effects with others in its class.

Life situation. A person who is being treated for end-stage cancer pain may have a very different treatment plan than a person with back pain who's still working and raising a family. The person with cancer pain may only be concerned about pain relief, whereas the latter person would need to balance pain relief with the ability to function in daily life.

Practical concerns. Many people need to consider the cost of their medication and the challenges of following a medication schedule. Some pain medications are short acting and have to be taken several times a day. Others have longer-lasting effects and can be taken less often.

Given all these factors, you and your doctor will choose medications that fit your particular needs. You might begin with low doses of medications that have fewer potential side effects. You and your doctor can then judge how this approach works before trying stronger medications, adding medications, or risking more side effects.

Getting the Best Results from Your Medications

According to the Agency for Healthcare Research and Quality, the most important step people can take to get the most from their medications is to take an active role in their health care. Some useful strategies are listed on pages 75 and 76.

Share information. It's essential that your doctor or doctors be aware of all the medications you're using, including any herbs, dietary supplements, vitamins, over-the-counter medicines, or complementary or alternative medicines. Your doctor needs to know the following information about your medications:

- The name of the medication (generic and brand names)
- Dosage: the amount and how often you take it
- Purpose: exactly why you are taking the medication
- How you take the medication: for example, whether you take it with or without food, in the morning, or just before going to bed
- Results: how well it seems to be working and whether there are side effects
- Other health conditions: for example, whether you're allergic to any medications, whether you're pregnant, or whether you have any other illnesses or conditions

Seek information. Read and keep the materials that come with your medicines. Ask your pharmacist or doctor for information that is specific to you. Know exactly why you're taking each medicine you have.

Stick to your plan. It is important to take your medicine exactly as directed. If you do change how you're taking your medicines or stop before they're gone, tell your doctor.

Talk to your doctor about changes. Your physical, mental, and emotional state can change over time. A medication that worked several months or years ago might have different effects on you today. Sometimes doses need to be changed. Pay attention to day-to-day changes in your health and report them to your doctor. (See appendix C, "Keeping a Journal.") Keep a list of questions you want to ask your doctor and bring it to your appointment. Don't be afraid to ask questions or to question any part of your treatment that doesn't seem to be working.

CHAPTER 5

Considering Complementary Medicine for Pain

During the past twenty years or so, some people seeking treatment for their ailments have looked beyond traditional medical doctors. They have turned to other groups of health care providers: men and women trained in complementary or alternative medicine (CAM). Initially, many who first turned to these therapies did so because traditional Western medicine had not provided the results they were seeking. Today, however, many people use CAM in conjunction with the care they receive from their doctor.

It's not unusual for people suffering with chronic pain to turn to other therapies as they look for relief. You may be considering this path as well, but with some concerns and questions. Are they safe? Will they work? Will they interfere with your current therapy and medications?

The National Center for Complementary and Alternative Medicine (NCCAM) is the federal government's lead agency for scientific research on CAM. NCCAM is dedicated to exploring complementary and alternative healing practices in the context of rigorous science, training CAM researchers, and disseminating authoritative information to the public and professionals.

There are many terms used to describe approaches to health care that are outside the realm of conventional medicine as practiced in the United States. In this chapter you'll find descriptions of some kinds of complementary and alternative medicine and suggestions on how to evaluate techniques that you may be considering.

What Is Complementary and Alternative Medicine?

Complementary and alternative medicine comprises diverse medical and health care systems, practices, and products that are not presently considered to be integral parts of conventional medicine. While scientific evidence exists regarding some CAM therapies, for others, key questions are yet to be answered through well-designed scientific studies—questions such as whether they are safe and whether they work for the diseases or medical conditions for which they are used.

The list of what is considered to be CAM changes continually, as those therapies that are proved to be safe and effective become adopted into conventional health care and as new approaches to health care emerge.

Complementary Medicine and Conventional Medicine: A Synergism

Today, more than one in three Americans are using complementary medicine, often in conjunction with conventional medicine. According to a nationwide government survey released in May 2004, 36 percent of U.S. adults aged eighteen years and over use some form of complementary medicine.[1]

We have seen that people experience pain in different ways. The same injury in two people doesn't necessarily produce the same pain response. Nor does the same pain therapy have the same effect for both. Synergism happens when the actions of two or more treatments have a greater effect together than you would expect to get by adding them together. In the case of pain control, when two or more treatments are combined, they provide a much more noticeable or dramatic effect than the sum of their individual effects. For example, massage and ice used separately might relieve the pain from a sprained wrist perhaps 10 percent each—a barely noticeable effect. But when combined, the treatments might yield 25 percent relief.

Synergism can take place when different approaches to pain management are used. It can happen when different medicines that work at different pain pathways are used together. It can happen when a medicine is used in conjunction with a physical technique such as massage or with nonpharmacological techniques such as meditation or acupuncture.

Communicating with Your Doctor about Complementary Therapies

You may be considering, or already using, complementary medicine for pain, but perhaps you're hesitant to talk to your doctor about these treatments because you're afraid he or she will automatically dismiss those options. While it's true that some doctors may not want to discuss such therapies, many doctors in the United States are now referring people to complementary medicine practitioners. Your doctor may, in fact, be very accepting of your decision and be happy to discuss these options with you.

Regardless of your doctor's opinion of complementary medicine, however, it's important to let him or her know what treatments you're using. By communicating carefully with your doctor, he or she can provide you with information about risks and benefits so that you can make informed decisions regarding these treatments.

Taking Responsibility for Your Health Care

You are the person who ultimately has the final say in your medical care. The better informed you are, the better decisions you can make. That's true whether you're deciding about traditional Western medicine or complementary medicine therapy. As we have pointed out before, you will fare much better if you take some responsibility for your progress and for your health care as a whole. We know that when patients take charge of their health and become well informed about their care—when they become partners with the medical staff who are helping them—they are more satisfied with their care and with its results. We encourage you to be a motivated and well-educated patient in pursuing nonpharmacological and complementary medicine techniques to help you achieve your goal of pain management without risk of addiction.

The following stories of Frank and Elena show how people dealing with chronic pain can learn about various therapies, weigh potential side effects, and choose a course of treatment that is appropriate for their situation.

Frank's Story

Frank was a very successful—and very busy—architect. "Too much time stooped over a drafting table," as he put it, had brought on chronic neck and arm pain. With the recommendation of his doctor, Frank had a relatively minor surgery for a damaged disk in his neck. After the surgery, he was pleased to find that his neck and arm pain were much improved, but to his dismay, he now had new pain in his upper back. Despite extensive tests and X-rays, his doctors were unable to find a cause for his pain, and as the weeks passed, Frank found that the pain increasingly interfered with his work. It gradually increased throughout the morning, and as a result, he would have to spend his lunch hour lying down. Once a week or so, he was unable to finish his regular workday.

Frank tried injections, physical therapy, and over-the-counter analgesics without satisfactory relief. He was reluctant to try stronger medications, particularly opioids, because he feared that they would cloud his thinking and interfere with his work. He was also concerned that his clients might lose confidence in him if they learned that he was taking strong, potentially addictive, medications for his pain.

His doctor recommended a pain specialist who in turn suggested to Frank that he consider some complementary therapies. Frank had learned Transcendental Meditation (TM) while in college, and this was the first technique he tried. He got a book from a local bookstore and reviewed its principles. Frank also discovered that his bookstore carried relaxation CDs that he could listen to while meditating. Frank then began to add a meditation session to his lunch hour rather than simply lying on his couch and feeling frustrated. He soon found that TM helped relieve some of the stress and muscle tension in his back. But unfortunately, his pain remained troublesome.

Frank then returned to his doctor, who added a weak opioid, tramadol, to his treatment plan, suggesting that Frank use it when the pain was at its worst in the afternoon. This suggestion alarmed Frank at first because he had been in recovery from alcohol and cocaine abuse for nearly twenty years, and he feared that an opioid might trigger a relapse. His doctor assured Frank that tramadol was a weak drug, which, if used carefully for pain relief, should not cause a problem. Both nevertheless agreed to set up a careful monitoring plan that involved Frank's family and his AA sponsor.

This step helped, but the pain remained a problem. Next, Frank searched the Internet and talked with friends about other complementary therapy techniques for pain. He decided that acupuncture was his best bet for pain control, and he returned to his pain specialist for a recommendation. The doctor sent him to another physician who was trained in both Western medicine and acupuncture. She performed about ten sessions of acupuncture.

At this point, Frank found that with both his complementary therapy techniques and his medication, he was able to manage his pain and remain productive in his job. However, the pain had limited his ability to exercise, and he was feeling out of shape. He also noticed that his posture at work exacerbated the pain. At the suggestion of a friend, he inquired at the local health club about tai chi and Pilates as ways to stay in shape and improve his posture. While he still has some problems with pain, Frank is able to work and exercise now. He hopes, in time, to stop taking tramadol altogether.

Elena's Story

Elena had been a fairly active woman for many years, but in her fifties, she had begun to experience pain from degenerative arthritis in her hips and knees. In part because she was in recovery, Elena wanted to try herbal dietary supplements first before turning to over-the-counter analgesics or stronger drugs.

After talking to friends with similar problems and searching the NCCAM Web site, she decided to try glucosamine and chondroitin sulfate. She went to a local health food and vitamin store and talked with staff there just to get another opinion. From what she'd been able to learn, she was unlikely to have any unwanted side effects from these two medications.

Just to be sure, however, Elena also went to her doctor to get more information about any supplements to avoid. She learned that various supplements can cause adverse reactions for people with certain medical problems. Because she'd had an ulcer three years earlier, Elena's doctor suggested that she might need to avoid NSAIDs. She agreed with Elena's choice of glucosamine and chondroitin sulfate, but suggested that Elena avoid feverfew, garlic, ginger, and ginkgo biloba because these can impair blood clotting. And because Elena had a history of substance abuse, she told her to avoid ephedra and ma huang because they can be subject to abuse, in addition to causing unsafe elevations in blood pressure.

Elena found that the glucosamine and chondroitin sulfate brought needed relief, though she also knew that at some point, she might be facing a decision about having a knee or hip replacement.

Commonly Used Complementary Medicine Therapies

Acupuncture. This method of healing developed in China at least three thousand years ago. Today, acupuncture describes a family of procedures involving stimulation of points on the body by a variety of techniques. American practices of acupuncture incorporate medical traditions from China, Japan, Korea, and other countries. The acupuncture technique that has been most studied scientifically involves penetrating the skin with thin, solid, metallic needles that are manipulated by the hands or by electrical stimulation. Considering it from a Western point of view, researchers now believe that acupuncture may increase levels of endogenous opioids, as well as modulating spinal cord processing of pain signals. Interestingly, acupuncture also works in animals and is a part of some veterinary medicine practices in the United States as well as in China.

Depending on their reasons for seeking acupuncture, patients may have one or several hair-thin needles inserted into their skin. Some go as deep as three inches, depending on where they're placed and the reason for the treatment. The needles usually are left in place for fifteen to thirty minutes. Patient and practitioner decide how many treatments will be needed and how often they'll take place.

Acupuncture is one of the most studied complementary medical practices, and it is gaining acceptance by Western medicine for treatment of certain conditions. A 1997 consensus statement released by the National Institutes of Health (NIH) stated that there is clear evidence that acupuncture helps relieve postoperative dental pain and that it's useful in treating nausea following surgery and chemotherapy. It may also be effective in stroke rehabilitation, headaches, menstrual cramps, tennis elbow, myofascial pain, osteoarthritis, low back pain, carpal tunnel syndrome, and asthma. It's most useful as part of a multidisciplinary approach to treating these conditions.

The results of using acupuncture for addiction have been inconclusive. A 2000 study published in the *Archives of Internal Medicine,* for example, indicated that acupuncture may aid in addiction treatment for cocaine abusers. Investigators at Yale University School of Medicine followed eighty-two cocaine-addicted participants who were randomly assigned to one of three groups. The first group received auricular acupuncture for addiction, which involves the insertion of needles into specific points in the outer ear. The second group received acupuncture in sites not known to give a therapeutic response, and the third received relaxation therapy only. The study found that more than half of the acupuncture patients (53.8 percent) were cocaine free after eight weeks, compared with one-quarter (23.5 percent) in the second group, and only 9.1 percent in the relaxation-therapy-only group.[2]

Acupuncture treatment for people with addiction problems is not new. It is most commonly used by those addicted to opioids, especially heroin, but is seeing increased use by those suffering from alcoholism. Many patients report that acupuncture helps reduce cravings for alcohol, aids in reducing withdrawal symptoms, and helps ease anxiety and depression. Some addicts on methadone maintenance use acupuncture to relieve nervousness and stress. It has also been a popular alternative or adjunct treatment for smoking cessation.

It's safe to conclude that even though it's questionable whether acupuncture can actually treat addiction, acupuncture itself is not addictive, and it's likely not going to make an addiction worse. It may be helpful for a variety of pain problems.

Acupressure. Another Chinese healing method, this technique involves applying pressure to the same points on the body used in acupuncture in order to relieve pain. Acupressure is said to relieve stress and tension; relax mind and body; increase blood circulation; provide relief from head, neck, and shoulder aches; promote the healing of injuries; and increase energy levels and an overall feeling of well-being.

Traditional Chinese medicine does not view acupressure as a separate system; the theory and practice of the points are essentially the same as in acupuncture. It's simply pressure at acupuncture points when needles are not available. Patients can therefore use it themselves.

Biofeedback. With this treatment technique, people are trained to improve their health by using signals from their own bodies. Specialists who provide biofeedback training range from psychiatrists and psychologists to dentists, internists, nurses, and physical therapists. Physical therapists use biofeedback to help stroke victims regain movement in weakened muscles. Psychologists use it to help tense and anxious clients learn to relax. Specialists in many different fields use biofeedback to help their patients cope with pain.

Biofeedback teaches people to use the mind to control the body. Through practice, you can learn to control your heart rate, skin temperature, blood pressure, and muscle tension, along with many other body functions. At a biofeedback session, your practitioner puts electrodes on your body and connects them to monitors. The monitors tell you muscle tension, temperature, heart rate, or other measures.

Patients usually are taught some form of relaxation exercise. Some learn to identify the circumstances that trigger their symptoms. They may also be taught how to avoid or cope with these stressful events. Most are encouraged to change their habits, and some are trained in special techniques for gaining such self-control.

Biofeedback is not magic. It cannot cure disease or, by itself, make a person healthy. It is a tool, one of many available to health care professionals, and it reminds physician and patient alike that behavior, thoughts, and feelings profoundly influence physical health.[3]

Chiropractic care. This treatment focuses on the relationship between bodily structure (primarily the spine) and function, and how that relationship affects the preservation and restoration of health. Chiropractors use manipulative therapy as an integral treatment tool. According to chiropractic theory, misaligned vertebrae can restrict your spine's range of motion and affect the nerves radiating from your spine. In turn, the organs that depend on those nerves may function improperly or become diseased. Chiropractic adjustments aim to realign your vertebrae and other joints.

Today, more and more chiropractors are combining standard chiropractic techniques with other therapies, such as exercise, acupuncture, or dietary and herbal supplements. Today, chiropractors sometimes work with medical doctors as part of a patient's medical team. Though they can't prescribe drugs or perform surgery, chiropractors may use some standard medical procedures. Studies indicate that spinal manipulation can effectively treat uncomplicated low back pain, especially if the pain has been present for less than one month.[4]

Dietary supplements. As defined by Congress in the Dietary Supplement Health and Education Act (DSHEA) of 1994, these are products, other than tobacco, taken by mouth that contain a "dietary ingredient" intended to supplement the diet. Dietary ingredients may include vitamins, minerals, herbs or other botanicals, amino acids, and substances such as enzymes, organ tissues, and metabolites. Dietary supplements come in many forms, including extracts, concentrates, tablets, capsules, gel caps, liquids, and powders. They have special requirements for labeling.

Herbal treatments aren't regulated nearly to the degree other drugs are, so little definitive proof exists about their effectiveness. Hundreds of herbs and supplements are available. If you decide to take an herbal supplement, purchase it from a reputable company, read the label carefully, and follow the directions for taking it.

It bears repeating that some herbal supplements contain ingredients that don't mix well with prescriptions or over-the-counter drugs, and others can increase the risk of bleeding during surgery. Keep track of whatever supplements you take and tell your doctor about them.[5]

Massage. One of the oldest, simplest forms of therapy, this is a system of stroking, pressing, and kneading different areas of the body to relieve pain and to relax, stimulate, and tone the body. Massage does much more than create a pleasant sensation on the skin; it also works on the soft tissues (the muscles, tendons, and ligaments) to improve blood flow. Although it largely affects those muscles just under the skin, its benefits may also reach the deeper layers of muscle and possibly even the organs themselves. Massage also stimulates blood circulation and assists the lymphatic system, which runs parallel to the circulatory system, improving the elimination of waste throughout the body.

Practitioners of massage describe the following benefits: it is relaxing, soothing, and healing. It eases tension, stiffness, and pain; improves breathing and circulation; and enhances well-being.

Although a single massage will be enjoyable, practitioners say that the effects of massage are cumulative and a course of massage treatments will bring the greatest benefit. Regular massage can have the effect of stretching and relaxing the entire body mechanism, thus helping prevent unnecessary strains and injuries that might otherwise occur due to excess tension. Massage can stimulate or calm the nervous system, depending upon what is required by the individual, and it can help reduce fatigue, leaving the receiver with a feeling of replenished energy. At its best, massage has the potential to restore the individual physically, mentally, and spiritually.

Meditation and prayer. These can also enhance the mind-body connection. The use of meditation for healing is not new. Meditative techniques are the product of diverse cultures and peoples around the globe; some are rooted in the world's oldest religious traditions. The value of meditation to alleviate suffering and promote healing has been known and practiced for thousands of years. It is one of the proven alternative therapies. The form called Transcendental Meditation has been validated by more than five hundred scientific studies at more than two hundred independent research institutions in thirty countries.[6]

More and more doctors are prescribing meditation as a way to lower blood pressure, improve exercise performance in people with angina, help people with asthma breathe easier, relieve insomnia, and generally relax the everyday stresses of life. Meditation is a safe way to balance a person's physical, emotional, and mental states. It is simple and can benefit everybody.

During a meditation session, people sit still and focus on something, maybe a word or their deep breathing. This is also called mindfulness, and it relaxes the body by slowing breathing and heart rate while also decreasing muscle tension. This deeply relaxed state can help people manage pain and reduce stress and anxiety.

Movement therapies. These include tai chi, qi gong, and the Alexander, Feldenkrais, and Trager methods, among others. These therapies espouse the philosophy that over time, or in response to injury or disease, people begin to hold and move their body in unhealthy patterns, causing stress and tension. Practitioners maintain that these therapies can help control pain and foster an overall sense of well-being. Exercises are designed to increase flexibility, improve posture, and facilitate healthy movement. Sometimes meditation and relaxation are included to help achieve these goals. Movement therapies may be particularly helpful for people suffering pain from musculoskeletal disorders or myofascial pain.

Naturopathic medicine. Also known as naturopathy, this complementary medical system is founded upon a holistic philosophy; it combines traditional therapies with the most current advances in modern medicine. Naturopathic medicine is used for the management of a broad range of health conditions, including pain.

Naturopathic medicine proposes that there is a healing power in the body that establishes, maintains, and restores health. Practitioners work with the patient with a goal of supporting this power, through treatments such as nutrition and lifestyle counseling, dietary supplements, medicinal plants, exercise, homeopathy, and treatments from traditional Chinese medicine.[7]

Osteopathic medicine. This form of conventional medicine emphasizes diseases arising in the musculoskeletal system. Osteopathy holds an underlying belief that all of the body's systems work together, and disturbances in one system may affect function elsewhere in the body. Some osteopathic physicians practice osteopathic manipulation: a full-body system of hands-on techniques to alleviate pain, restore function, and promote health and well-being.

Most doctors of osteopathy (DOs) combine conventional Western medicine (drugs and surgery) with specific manipulative techniques taught in the osteopathic medical colleges. Osteopathic medical training focuses on preventive care with a special emphasis on the musculoskeletal system. Because their medical degree and license are recognized as the equivalent of those of a medical doctor (MD) in the United States, DOs can utilize all recognized diagnostic and therapeutic methods in their practices.[8]

Traditional Chinese medicine. Also known as TCM, this is the current name for an ancient system of health care from China. TCM is based on a concept of balanced *chi,* the vital energy that is believed to flow throughout the body. Chi regulates a person's spiritual, emotional, mental, and physical balance and is said to be influenced by the opposing forces of *yin* (negative energy) and *yang* (positive energy). Disease is thought to result from disruptions in the flow of chi and from an imbalance of yin and yang. Among the components of TCM are herbal and nutritional therapy, restorative physical exercises, meditation, acupuncture, and remedial massage.[9]

Yoga. This ancient art is a practical aid, not a religion. It's based on a harmonizing system of development for the body, mind, and spirit that uses postures and meditation to enhance the mind-body connection. Practitioners of yoga view it as a comprehensive approach to health and fitness that can increase energy, strength, aerobic capacity, and flexibility. Done regularly, yoga provides effective stress management by fostering positive thought patterns and using deep relaxation techniques.

A typical yoga session incorporates four elements: breathing, relaxation, poses, and meditation. Many poses exist, and each is intended for a specific purpose, such as improving strength or posture or relaxing organs. At the same time, yoga encourages you to focus on your movements, which relaxes the body and clears the mind.[10]

Finding Reliable Information about Complementary Medicine Therapies

If you are interested in a complementary medicine therapy, do some research. Learn what scientific studies have discovered about it; avoid choosing a therapy simply on the basis of an advertisement, a Web site, or anecdotal evidence. Understanding a treatment's risks, potential benefits, and scientific evidence is critical to your health and safety. Scientific research on many complementary medicine therapies is relatively new, so this kind of information may not be available for every therapy. However, many studies on complementary medicine treatments are under way, including those that the National Center for Complementary and Alternative Medicine (NCCAM) supports, and our knowledge and understanding of complementary medicine is increasing all the time.

One way to find scientifically based information is to talk to your health care practitioners. Tell them about the therapy you are considering and ask any questions you may have about safety, effectiveness, or interactions with prescription or nonprescription medications. They may know about the therapy and be able to advise you on its safety and use. If your practitioner can't answer your questions, he or she may be able to refer you to someone who can. Your practitioner may also be able to help you interpret the results of scientific articles you have found.

Use the Internet to search medical libraries and databases for information (see appendix E). CAM on PubMed, the complementary and alternative medicine database developed by NCCAM and the National Library of Medicine, gives citations or brief summaries of the results of scientific studies on complementary medicine (www.nlm.nih.gov/nccam/camonpubmed.html). In some cases, it provides links to publishers' Web sites, where you may be able to view or obtain the full articles. The articles cited in CAM on PubMed are peer reviewed; that is, other scientists in the same field have reviewed the article, the data, and the conclusions and judged them to be accurate and important to the field. The Directory of Information Resources Online (DIRLINE), compiled by the National Library of Medicine (dirline.nlm.nih.gov), is another good site.

For information on dietary supplements, turn to medical libraries or to Web-based resources such as PubMed (www. ncbi.nlm.nih.gov/entrez/) and the Food and Drug Administration (FDA) site (www.cfsan.fda.gov/). Another database, International Bibliographic Information on Dietary Supplements, is useful for searching the scientific literature on herbs and other dietary supplements (www.ods.od.nih.gov/databases /ibids.html). Information specifically about dietary supplements can be found on the FDA's Center for Food Safety and Applied Nutrition Web site at www.cfsan.fda.gov. Or visit the FDA's Web page on recalls and safety alerts at www. fda.gov/opacom/7alerts.html. Another useful resource is the Diet, Health, and Fitness Consumer Information site at www. ftc.gov/bcp/menu-health.htm.

Evaluating Web Site Reputability

The number of Web sites offering health-related resources grows every day. Many sites provide valuable information, while others may have information that is unreliable or misleading.

Any good health-related Web site should make it easy for you to learn who is responsible for the site and its information. You should know how the site pays for itself. The source of a Web site's funding should be clearly stated or readily apparent. For example, Web addresses ending in ".gov" denote a federal government–sponsored site. Does it sell advertising?

Is it sponsored by a drug company? The source of funding can affect what content is presented, how it is presented, and what the site owners want to accomplish on the site.

Many health and medical sites post information collected from other Web sites or sources. If the person or organization in charge of the site did not create the information, the original source should be clearly labeled. In addition to identifying who wrote the material you are reading, the site should describe the evidence on which the material is based. Medical facts and figures should have references, such as to articles in medical journals. Also, opinions or advice should be clearly set apart from information that is "evidence-based," that is, based on research results. Is there an editorial board? Do people with excellent professional and scientific qualifications review the material before it is posted?

Web sites should be reviewed and updated on a regular basis. It is particularly important that medical information be current. The most recent update or review date should be clearly posted. Even if the information has not changed, you want to know whether the site owners have reviewed it recently to ensure that it is still valid.

Read and understand any privacy policy or similar language on the site, and don't sign up for anything that you are not sure you fully understand. There should always be a way for you to contact the site owner if you have problems, questions, or feedback. If the site hosts chat rooms or other online discussion areas, it should tell visitors what the terms of using this service are. Is it moderated? If so, by whom, and why? It is always a good idea to spend time reading the discussion without joining in, so that you feel comfortable with the environment before becoming a participant.[11]

The Safety of Complementary Medicine Therapies

As with any therapy, there can be risks with complementary medicine treatments. Ask about the risks, benefits, and alternatives before agreeing to try any therapy. If you have more than one health care provider, let all of them know about the complementary medicine and conventional therapies you are using. This will help each provider ensure that all aspects of your health care work together.

Keep some general issues in mind, too, in regard to product labeling and potential interactions. Many consumers believe, for example, that "natural" means the same thing as "safe." This is not necessarily true. For example, think of mushrooms that grow in the wild: some are safe to eat, while others are poisonous. For a complementary medicine product that is sold over the counter (without a prescription), such as a dietary supplement, safety can also depend on the product's components or ingredients, the origin of those ingredients, and the quality of the manufacturing process, for example, whether steps have been taken to prevent contamination.

Dietary supplement ingredients sold in the United States before October 15, 1994, are not required to be reviewed by the FDA for their safety before they are marketed because they are presumed safe based on their history of use by humans. Manufacturers do not have to provide the FDA with evidence that dietary supplements are effective or safe; however, they are not permitted to market proven unsafe or ineffective products. Once a dietary supplement is marketed, the FDA has to prove that the product is not safe in order to restrict its use or remove it from the market. In contrast, before being allowed to market a drug product, pharmaceutical manufacturers must obtain FDA approval by providing convincing evidence that it is both safe and effective.

Herbal or botanical products and other dietary supplements may interact with prescription or nonprescription medications. They may also have negative, even dangerous, effects on their own. Research has shown that the herb St. John's wort, for example, which is used by some people to treat depression, may cause certain drugs to become less effective. Kava, an herb that has been used for insomnia, stress, and anxiety, has been linked to liver damage. Ginseng can increase the stimulant effects of caffeine (such as in coffee, tea, and cola). It can also lower blood sugar levels, creating the possibility of problems when used with diabetes drugs. Ginkgo biloba, taken with anticoagulant or antiplatelet drugs, can increase the risk of bleeding. It may also interact with certain psychiatric drugs and with certain drugs that affect blood sugar levels.

The active ingredient(s) in many herbs and herbal supplements are not known. There may be dozens, even hundreds, of such compounds in an herbal supplement. Scientists are currently working to identify these ingredients and analyze products. Published analyses of herbal supplements have found differences between what's listed on the label and what's in the bottle. This means that you may be taking less— or more—of the supplement than what the label indicates. Moreover, the word "standardized" on a product label is no guarantee of higher product quality, since in the United States there is no legal definition of "standardized" (or "certified" or "verified") for supplements.

Some herbal supplements have been found to be contaminated with metals, unlabeled prescription drugs, microorganisms, or other substances. There has been an increase in the number of Web sites that sell and promote herbal supplements on the Internet. The federal government has taken legal action against a number of company sites because they have been shown to contain incorrect statements and to be deceptive to consumers.[12]

Evaluating Claims about Effectiveness of Complementary Medicine Therapies

Statements that manufacturers and providers of complementary medicine therapies may make about the therapy's effectiveness and other benefits can sound reasonable and promising. However, they may not be backed up by scientific evidence. Before you begin using a complementary medicine treatment, it is a good idea to ask if there is scientific evidence, not just personal stories, to back up the claims. Ask the manufacturer or the practitioner for scientific articles or the results of studies. They should be willing to share this information, if it exists. Visit the FDA online at www.fda.gov to look for information about the product or practice. Check with the Federal Trade Commission (FTC) at www.ftc.gov for any fraudulent claims or consumer alerts regarding the therapy.

How does the provider or manufacturer describe the treatment? The FDA advises that certain types of language may sound impressive but actually disguise a lack of science. Be wary of terminology such as "innovation," "quick" or "miracle" cure, "exclusive product," "magical" or "new" discovery. Watch out for claims of a "secret formula." If a therapy were a cure for a disease, it would be widely reported and prescribed or recommended. Legitimate scientists want to share their knowledge so that their peers can review their data. Be suspicious of phrases like "suppressed by government" or claims that the medical profession or research scientists have conspired to prevent a therapy from reaching the public. Finally, be wary of claims that a therapy cures a wide range of unrelated diseases, for example, cancer, diabetes, and AIDS. No product can treat every disease and condition.

Selecting a Complementary Medicine Practitioner

Selecting a health care practitioner—for conventional or complementary medicine—is an important decision and can be key to ensuring that you are receiving the best health care. The information below will help you answer frequently asked questions about selecting a complementary medicine practitioner, issues to consider when making your decision, and important questions to ask the practitioner you select.

Remember, conventional medicine is practiced by holders of MD (medical doctor) or DO (doctor of osteopathy) degrees and by their allied health professionals, such as physical therapists, psychologists, and registered nurses. Other terms for conventional medicine include *allopathy, Western, mainstream, orthodox,* and *regular medicine.* Some of these practitioners are also practitioners of CAM.

If you are seeking a complementary medicine practitioner, speak with your current health care provider(s) or someone you believe to be knowledgeable about your area of interest. Ask for a recommendation for the type of practitioner you are seeking. Make a list of complementary medicine practitioners and gather information about each before making your first visit. Ask basic questions about their credentials and practice. Where did they receive their training? What licenses or certifications do they have?

Consider cost. Few complementary medicine therapies are covered by insurance, and when they are, the amount of coverage offered varies depending upon the insurer. Before agreeing to a treatment that a complementary medicine practitioner suggests, ask your insurer whether any portion of the cost will be covered.

After you select a practitioner, make a list of questions to ask at your first visit, including the risks, benefits, and alternatives of the proposed therapy. You may want to bring a friend or family member to help you ask questions and note answers. Afterward, assess the visit and decide whether the practitioner is right for you. Did you feel comfortable? Could the practitioner answer your questions and respond to you in a way that satisfied you? Does the treatment plan seem reasonable and acceptable to you?

If you are not satisfied or comfortable, you can look for a different practitioner or stop treatment. However, as with any conventional treatment, talk with your practitioner first to make sure that it is safe to simply stop. It may not be advisable to stop some therapies midway through a course of treatment.

Discuss with your practitioner the reasons you are not satisfied or comfortable with treatment. If you decide to stop a therapy or seek another practitioner, share this information with any other health care practitioners you may have, as this will help them make decisions about your care. Communicating with your practitioner can be key to ensuring the best possible health care.

Though long viewed with suspicion by medical doctors, complementary medicine has been embraced by an ever-growing number of people. Today, many of these techniques are being provided by CAM practitioners in medical clinics side-by-side with medical doctors. A February 28, 2005, *Time Magazine* cover story on treating pain documented the ways in which medical clinics and leading pain-management centers nationwide are embracing "holistic healing" techniques and drawing on a full range of options, from ibuprofen and acupuncture to stress management, vitamins, and imaging techniques. We now know that, despite what many have long believed, it takes more than a prescription to treat pain.

CHAPTER 6

Winning Ways to Cope with Pain

Living well with pain isn't just about taking steps to control your pain. It involves paying attention to and caring for your overall health, so that you can enjoy life to its fullest.

The goal of this book is to give you as many tools as possible for dealing with pain. To avoid the potential for triggering relapse for people in recovery, we're limiting one significant tool in your toolbox by recommending opioids only under very specific and controlled conditions. Because of this limitation, it's all the more important that you be familiar with all the other tools available and have them at your disposal.

In chapters 4 and 5, we gave you a number of alternatives for addressing chronic pain by introducing you to traditional and complementary medicine techniques. In chapter 1, we presented information about the emotional and psychological components of pain. In this chapter, you'll learn more about psychological and behavioral techniques for pain control. The material here and in chapter 5 are closely related in that they both address a similar problem: how to ease acute and chronic pain with fewer medications and, if possible, without the use of opioids.

In the throes of addiction, people often take extreme measures to avoid or eliminate pain, be it physical, emotional, or psychological. To then find themselves in chronic pain during recovery can be very difficult psychologically. For this reason, it's important to recognize that chronic pain can be a very powerful relapse trigger.

Psychological and Behavioral Techniques for Pain Control

Psychological or behavioral therapies that address pain are designed principally to improve function, regardless of pain. This approach in a sense says, "Yes, we know you have pain, but just for now, we're going to focus more on what you *can* do and *how* you're going to approach your daily living activities." This is very much a behavioral approach that may involve learning coping and stress-reduction techniques, as well as examining your attitudes about your overall life situation. Even if the pain can't be eliminated, there are still a number of changes people can make in their attitude about their situation and in their behavior to make their lives much better.

The physical nonpharmacological approach to controlling pain is still similar to a drug-based approach in that it is designed to *relieve* pain. It does not address means by which you can *cope* with pain. There is, however, an overlap between the two areas. Some stress-reduction techniques, for example, can both relieve physiological pain and help a person cope psychologically with chronic pain.

In a sense, it is somewhat arbitrary to make the distinction between the physical and psychological approaches. In day-to-day life, we encourage people to use both approaches in concert. It's not necessary to do everything you can to relieve the pain and then, when you can't get any further relief, turn to psychological approaches to handle the pain that remains. Creating such a split is not particularly wise or effective. That approach can actually be counterproductive. Some people, for example, never move on to try the psychological approaches because they have become fixated on the pain that remains after drug therapy.

Ideally, if you want to deal with acute or chronic pain, and especially if you want to avoid opioid medications for a serious pain problem, explore and use all the tools you have available: both physiological and psychological. You may not need all of them. Some may neither interest nor work for you. That's why our approach is to introduce you to as many tools as we can and to encourage you to find the ones that work well for *you*. Adopting a healthier lifestyle can help you stay active and productive, feel good about yourself, effectively address your pain concerns—and support your recovery.

The Pain-Stress Cycle

Life itself can be a challenge, and we can view pain as just one of many events that can throw a roadblock in our path. What's more, pain and stress go hand in hand. When you're in pain, the stresses of daily life can become more challenging. Small problems or hassles turn into major ones. Stress may also cause you to do things that worsen your pain: tensing your muscles, tightening your shoulders, clenching your teeth. This is the pain-stress cycle: pain causes stress, and stress intensifies pain.

The first step in breaking this pain-stress cycle is to realize that stress is *your response* to a situation, not the situation itself. Therefore, it's something you can control. That's why events that are stressful for you may not bother your spouse or friends. For example, your walk from your car to your office may leave you anxious and tense because you worry while you walk. Your colleague, however, finds his walk a relaxing time to get a little exercise and enjoy being outside. Understanding that you *do* have control over your stress can help you develop positive strategies for dealing with stress.

Responding to Stress

When you encounter stress, your body responds in a manner similar to a physical threat. It automatically prepares to face a perceived challenge. This "fight-or-flight response," as it's commonly known, results from a release of hormones that prompts a number of physical reactions: faster heart rate, increased blood pressure, and faster and shallower breathing. Your facial muscles tighten and your body perspires more.

Stress can be negative or positive. Positive stress provides a feeling of excitement and opportunity. It often helps athletes perform better in competition than in practice, for example. Negative stress occurs when you feel out of control or under constant or intense pressure. You may have trouble concentrating or sleeping, or you may feel alone. Family, finances, work, isolation, and health problems, including pain, are common causes of negative stress.

Living in a constant state of stress can negatively affect your health. In addition to the strain it puts on your cardiovascular system, the hormone cortisol released during stress may depress your immune system, making you more susceptible to infection and disease.

What Are Your Triggers?

Stress is often associated with situations or events that you find difficult to handle. It is worth asking yourself what situations trigger the stress. Take some time to think about it. Your stress may be linked to external factors, such as family, work, relationships, raising children, and so on. It may also rise from internal factors such as poor health habits, negative attitudes and feelings, and unrealistic expectations or goals.

Make a list of what seem to be sources of stress for you. Then ask yourself what you can do to lessen or avoid them. Some stressors you can control and some you can't, so concentrate on the ones you can change.

You can also try setting some *moderate* goals for yourself; moderation is a key concept here. *Moderate* means making sure that you're making *reasonable* progress—not too fast and not too slow. Don't overdo an activity or effort one day only to pay the price the next. Try to avoid wide swings between overactivity and inactivity. The aim is to balance activities, goals, and expectations.

Lifestyle Choices to Control Pain

Lifestyle and attitude choices can help you reduce the stressors you can control, and better live with the ones you can't. A rewarding life is possible even with chronic pain. A positive outlook and a willingness to explore various coping options can boost your success. Cultivate these habits:

Exercise regularly. Physical activity for thirty minutes daily relieves emotional stress, maintains muscle tone and stamina, controls weight, and helps prevent problems such as diabetes, high blood pressure, and heart disease.

Get enough sleep. Consistent bedtimes and wake-up times may help you sleep more soundly. Avoid napping during the day if it's likely to disrupt your sleep at night. Practicing stress-reduction techniques can help you sleep better, despite the pain you may have.

Eat well. With a nutritious diet keeping your body systems working well, you're better able to control stress and pain.

Plan your day. A daily schedule gives you more control of your life. Prioritize and pace yourself. Learn to delegate tasks and say no to added commitments if you're not up to them. Do your daily tasks efficiently, but be realistic about the time they'll take.

Take breaks. Remember, you don't have to be productive every minute. Take time to relax, stretch, or walk periodically during the day.

Get organized. Organize your home and work space to reduce physical and mental clutter. Talk with an occupational therapist about tools and techniques to ease tasks such as dressing or household chores. Stay on top of preventive maintenance for your home and car to prevent untimely or stressful repairs.

Avoid unnecessary medications. Wean yourself from the medicines you don't need.

Identify and use your capabilities. Keep your skills and talents alive—even if you're functioning within limits.

Stay connected to others. Seek out caring friends and relatives and communicate regularly with them. Join support groups with others experiencing similar problems. Understand and express the feelings that pain creates, but don't dwell on the pain itself. If you are in recovery, consider boosting your Twelve Step meeting attendance and "working the Steps." If you can't get out, bring a meeting to your home. Talk regularly with peers and sponsors about addressing pain and other stressors. Ask for help when you need it, and if others suggest that you need help, act on their advice. Don't fall prey to the idea that you can, or should, do everything on your own. Stay in touch.

Be patient. Your health may improve slowly; adjusting to loss and accepting change may also take time. Practice patience to reduce anxiety and stress.

Relief through Relaxation

It's impossible to avoid all sources of stress, but you *can* change how you react to these situations by practicing relaxation techniques. Relaxation can help relieve the stress that aggravates chronic pain. It also helps prevent muscle spasms and reduces muscle tension. Keep in mind, too, that learning to relax takes time. Don't get yourself stressed by your efforts to become less stressed!

Relaxation won't cure your pain, but it can

- reduce anxiety and conserve energy
- increase your self-control when dealing with stress
- help you recognize the difference between tense muscles and relaxed ones
- help you handle your daily demands
- help you remain alert, energetic, and productive

There are many ways to relax, so try a few and pick the ones that work best for you.

Deep breathing. Proper breathing is essential for good mental and physical health. Unlike children, most adults breathe from the chest: when they inhale their chest expands, when they exhale it contracts. Children, however, generally breathe from the diaphragm, the muscle that separates the chest from the abdomen (stomach). Their abdomen relaxes out with each inhalation. Deep breathing from the diaphragm, which adults can relearn, is relaxing. The next time you feel a surge of stress, try a few moments of deep breathing. Sit in a comfortable position and take deep, measured breaths by inhaling while counting up from one to four, pausing briefly, then exhaling while counting down from four to one. Do this twenty to thirty times and you're sure to feel refreshed. Be careful, though, not to tense muscles near your pain sites.

Progressive relaxation. This technique reduces muscle tension and can also relieve anxiety. To achieve deep muscle relaxation, gradually tense your muscles as tight as you can for about five seconds, then release the tension rapidly and let them go totally limp. Begin with the muscles in your hands, then move progressively to your arms, shoulders, and neck. Then move to your feet and work gradually up to your head. When you're finished, your muscles should be very relaxed and free of tension.

Guided imagery. If you think anxious thoughts, you become tense. You can use the power of your imagination to refocus your mind on positive, healing images. Take a comfortable position, close your eyes, and visualize a scene or place that you associate with safety and relaxation. It doesn't matter what you visualize, as long as it's calming to you. Try to experience the setting with all of your senses, as if you were actually there. For instance, imagine walking through a peaceful park. Picture the beautiful blue sky, smell the fresh air, hear the birds singing, and feel the warm breeze on your skin. The messages your brain receives as you imagine these senses help you relax. As you relax your mind, your body also relaxes.[1]

Prayer and meditation. These are an integral part of Twelve Step programs, and they are often used in complementary medicine therapies as well, as noted in chapter 5. One simple meditation technique is word repetition. Choose a word or phrase that cues you to relax, and then repeat it to yourself continuously. While doing so, breathe deeply and slowly and imagine something that gives you pleasant sensations of warmth and heaviness. When your mind wanders, simply bring it back to your word or image, and stay "in the moment." Other approaches include Mindfulness Meditation, as described in Jon Kabat-Zinn's book *Full Catastrophe Living* (see www.umassmed.edu/cfm); Transcendental Meditation (TM) (see www.tm.org); and Vipassana Meditation (see www.dhamma.org).

Emotional Awareness

Living with pain, particularly with chronic pain, brings up a variety of feelings—natural emotions that inevitably arise with any such disability or challenge. The loss of some degree of independence or the ability to pursue certain activities, even if only temporary, can elicit feelings of loss and grief similar to what we would feel at the loss of a person we love. It's helpful to acknowledge that this is a stressful event and can cause a major emotional crisis.

Some emotions you may experience include denial, disbelief, confusion, shock, sadness, depression, grief, yearning, anger, and despair. These feelings are normal and common reactions to loss. You may not be prepared for the intensity and duration of your emotions or how swiftly your moods may change. Be assured, however, that these feelings are healthy and appropriate and will help you come to terms with your situation.

Remember that it takes time to fully absorb the impact of any loss. Let yourself express whatever you're feeling. If need be, seek professional assistance to help work through your concerns. It's a sign of strength, not weakness, to seek help.

"Rethinking" Pain: Cognitive Behavioral Therapy

Chronic pain can cause people to cut back on their activities and social interactions, which can lead to loss of physical stamina and increased isolation. Such a combination of events can lead to depression. A vicious cycle results when physical, social, and emotional deterioration leads to more pain. You can learn to manage the pain so that it's not the main focus of your attention. This will help you concentrate on things in your life that give you pleasure or satisfaction and help you break the bad cycles.

Chronic pain can cause people to fall into a series of cognitive "mistakes"—mistakes in thinking that can lead them to become their own worst enemy. Cognitive behavioral therapy is an approach that can help people escape from these negative and often self-limiting thinking traps. The cognitive aspect involves using the rational mind and educational tools to achieve a goal, and the behavioral aspect denotes a strict focus on the actions taken and the results of those actions. This approach involves learning to recognize and think your way out of vicious emotional cycles and seek alternatives when you encounter roadblocks.

It's essential to be as positive as you can when addressing chronic pain. Avoiding negative self-talk can be difficult, but spending time with people who have a positive outlook and a sense of humor can help. In fact, laughter actually helps ease pain: it helps your body release endorphins, the brain chemicals that give you pain relief and a sense of well-being.

Addressing and resolving negative thinking patterns is crucial because those patterns affect the whole cycle of pain and disability in patients who have chronic pain. These "errors" in thinking and behavior often lead to less activity. The less active you are, the worse you'll likely feel, because you may become frustrated or angry. In addition, your body may start to lose muscle tone and aerobic conditioning. As a result, you may actually have increased pain because you're not exercising, stretching, or doing other rehabilitation activities.

Cognitive behavioral therapy offers another effective means of approaching and coping with pain and breaking this cycle.

If you let it, the rational side of your mind can exert control over, or at least provide perspective on, your emotional side. When people are trying to live with pain, and in particular with chronic pain, it's not unusual to fall into some unproductive or even negative thinking patterns. Cognitive behavioral therapy provides effective techniques to deal with flawed ways of thinking. Such problem thought patterns include the following.

Filtering. With this thinking pattern, people tend to focus on the negative aspects of their lives while filtering out positive aspects. A person with chronic low back pain might say to himself, in effect, "When my back hurts, there is *nothing* in my life that is positive." That's filtering because, of course, there are some positive aspects to his life. He can still enjoy reading, he has a loving family, he can still do some of his favorite activities, but he is actually choosing not to recognize those positive aspects.

Polarized thinking. Here, people see the world in absolutes: everything is either all good or all bad, positive or negative. For example, a person with leg pain that prevents her from walking very much might say to herself, "Well, I can't walk my normal amount, so I won't walk at all." Taking a more moderate or balanced view of her life would allow her to set intermediate goals.

Overgeneralizing. A person with this thought pattern might say to himself, "My pain ruined my last social event, so all social activities will be miserable for me." By learning to look at such events more rationally, he would see that while there are times when his pain limits him, there are other times when it doesn't. He could also learn to recognize when his pain would spoil a particular activity and when it wouldn't.

Catastrophizing. This is "what if" thinking in negative form, "making a mountain out of a molehill." A person with chronic pain might say to herself, "I can't go out with my friends because if my pain acts up, everything will be ruined." As a result, she stops going out.

Mind reading. A pain sufferer might believe she knows what others are feeling and why they act as they do—especially toward her. "My friends don't want me to be around them," she might assume, but her friends may not be thinking this at all.

The "shoulds." Chronic pain can be limiting. Rather than learning to focus on what they can still do, some people regularly tell themselves that they "should" do tasks that are problems for them. For example, "I should work in the garden because the weeds are growing" or "I should really dust all those shelves" or "I should go watch my son's Little League game." People stuck in the "shoulds" continually make mental lists of what activities they ought to accomplish rather than making a reasonable list of activities that they really *want* to do.

The martyr syndrome. Some people view life as a cosmic balance scale wherein they expect sacrifices and self-denial to pay off in some positive way. They may see their problem with chronic pain as some kind of cosmic bad luck or retribution: "Why do I have to suffer like this?" or "What good is going to come from having to deal with this pain?" With this kind of thinking, people begin to lose a realistic perspective on their problems.

Recognizing Negative Approaches to Pain

It's so easy and all too common to fall into cycles of seeing only what you can't do rather than what you can do. And this is understandable because filtering, polarized thinking, and the like are natural ways of reacting to a situation. They're defense mechanisms, and as such, they are often unconscious and hard to recognize. You can do a lot on your own, to be sure, but you may find that you need help, too. You might consider the following strategies:

- Talk to an objective third party such as a counselor or a psychologist.
- Read self-help books for people coping with chronic pain.
- Join a self-help or support group of people facing a similar challenge, and discuss your situation with your current recovery group. In addition to providing support and camaraderie, they can help you find other resources and learn about other positive ways to approach your problem.

Everyone is subject to thinking fallacies to some degree, whether in response to chronic pain or simply to the daily challenges of life. If you are in recovery, you are likely familiar with dysfunctional and negative thinking patterns. Whether you have the extra burden of substance abuse or not, such thinking seems to be part of the human condition.

It's easy to imagine someone saying to herself, "You know, I've got all these challenges, so I need a drink" or "I'm dealing with all this trouble, so I have to take a pain pill." A better approach would be to say, "Well, let's take a step back. Maybe there are other ways I could handle this problem with pain."

People who have gone through a Twelve Step program may, in fact, be ahead of the game in that they are already familiar with these techniques and with the tremendous value of support groups. These techniques can be applied to the challenge of pain just as they have been applied to the challenge of dealing with stressors in the context of addiction and recovery.

Secondary Gains Associated with Chronic Pain

For some people, maintaining a state of chronic pain can have positive outcomes. For example, someone who's living alone and often feels lonely may look forward to the attention he or she receives as a result of chronic pain. Friends and neighbors come to visit. Home care providers stop by regularly. Appointments with a doctor or physical therapist are opportunities to get out and interact with others who care. People who are on leave from a job they greatly dislike and who receive worker's compensation may decide that they have a vested interest in staying incapacitated. Such secondary gain, even if unconscious, can affect the outcome of chronic pain treatment. It is usually best to resolve legal and insurance issues as quickly as possible, so you can move on with the rest of your life.

The Pain Cycle and Anger, Depression, and Relationships

These psychological aspects can dramatically affect pain, though they are all too often ignored, even by the medical community. If a patient tells his doctor, "My back hurts," he may get a fairly stock response: a recommendation of muscle relaxants and pain medication. That may be an adequate answer for a person with an acute problem, but what if the pain is actually a symptom of an underlying behavioral or personal problem? Expanding on this example, let's say that the painkillers didn't work. The patient goes back to his doctor two more times, and finally the doctor catches on and says, "Maybe this pain is not just a back problem. Maybe it's a symptom of some underlying issues." Doctor and patient talk, and it turns out that the patient hasn't been sleeping well for months. He's having ongoing problems with his employer, and because of some changes at work, he now hates his job but can't quit because he needs the money. Lately his wife and children have become frustrated with his negative attitude. His back pain has been brought on through muscle tension as a result of his personal problems.

People who have experienced abuse or post-traumatic stress disorder (PTSD) at some point in their lives are more likely to suffer from chronic pain. Such experiences can also contribute to a person's chronic pain response. Why this is so is not clear, but research nevertheless shows that many people find that their chronic pain lessens once they begin to address those traumatic experiences.

This is *not* to say, however, that the pain is "all in a person's head." The way we think and our emotional state affect our physical well-being, just as our physical state affects our emotional state and our thinking patterns. It's not a matter of which came first, "the chicken or the egg." You may actually have something wrong with your back. You may actually have a bad job and a troubled marriage. And when the physical and psychological aspects come together, they can build on each other without your conscious awareness. In addressing these factors, however, it's not wise to simply try to convince yourself that you don't have pain because "there's not really a physical problem."

On the contrary, it's important to recognize that there are both positive and negative ways to live with pain. You have the power to choose the approach you're going to take. Cognitive and behavioral techniques offer a functional, adaptive, and positive way to live with pain. Often people who apply these techniques find incidentally that their pain is better, or at least that it doesn't bother them as much.

Imagine, for a moment, that you had a terrible migraine that had lasted several days. You would have two choices. You could lie in bed and think of nothing but your pain, growing more and more frustrated by the fact that you are missing work and other activities. Or you could acknowledge that you have a terrible headache but decide to try, somehow, to make some modest progress toward a small goal. With the latter choice, you could accomplish something despite the migraine—not at your normal capacity, of course, but you could retain some control over your life.

The following story illustrates this kind of approach.

Paula's Story

I'd been having some problems with back pain for some time. I'd gone to my family doctor, who prescribed some pain medications. I started out with ibuprofen, which only helped a little. Eventually I ended up taking oxycodone (OxyContin). I really, really wanted to get rid of this back pain. I knew from some scans that I had some bulging disks, and I had been told that there was also some inflammation back there and possibly a pinched nerve. I thought maybe I should have surgery, but the doctors I went to didn't agree. I guess they were being conservative, but I was getting frustrated. I kept wondering if surgery would help.

After some time on the drugs, my life just started unraveling. I was on worker's comp disability, and my employer and the insurance companies were fighting with each other over that. No one wanted to pay, of course. The pain was getting worse. I kept having bad days, and the whole situation seemed stuck. Nothing was happening. I just kept getting really ticked off, and then I'd get into a funk where I couldn't keep up with the housework, and of course my husband was getting frustrated with me because of all this trouble.

Eventually, I had a really bad day. I had my husband drive me to a very good medical center. I had looked up the name of its pain specialist, so I went straight to her and said, "The first thing I need is my prescription refilled, and the second thing I need is to find a surgeon who will fix my back once and for all."

But that's not what happened. Right away she asked me to take a couple of deep breaths and try to relax. Then she wanted to hear my story, and not just about my back pain. We talked in great detail about how my life had been limited, about my frustrations and other feelings, and about the problems with my employer. She helped me see how angry I was, and how I'd been spending a lot of time fighting with insurance companies and Social Security staff. We talked, too, about how the housework and chores and shopping were not getting done and how my husband was trying to help with some of that.

She helped me look at some stuff that was going on that I never really paid attention to—or at least that I didn't think was related to my back pain. First off, I'd been sleeping poorly for months. During the day, I didn't have much to do—actually, I couldn't do much, or so I thought—so I tended to watch TV most of the afternoon, nodding and dozing a bunch. Of course, that wasn't helping my sleeping problems at all. I wasn't tired at night, so I'd lie there awake because the house was quiet and there was nothing to distract me from the pain in my back.

Next, she asked me to think about just how much the medications actually helped me, whether they'd actually made it easier for me to do my housework, get around in the car, and so on. And when I actually looked at that, I had to say, "No, they haven't helped very much."

After listening to my problems, she was quiet for a bit. Then she made a suggestion that really surprised me. She asked if I'd be willing to try a different approach—not with more or different medications, but by trying to move on now and look at ways to live better with the pain rather than being stuck where I was, just trying to cure it. I broke down a bit at that point, because it made me realize that everything I'd been doing wasn't really working. But I was scared, too, that maybe she meant I should just give up, that nothing would get better, and that I'd just be stuck watching TV all day.

Well, I was really wrong about that! At our next appointment, we sat down and looked at a list of moderate goals she'd asked me to create. Our first and main goal was to try to get the worker's comp case settled so the financial problems could finally be put to rest. Then she helped me look at taking a more meaningful approach to my life. She helped me see that I was looking at life as an "all or none" situation. Sure, there were some things I couldn't do like before, but there was a lot I could still do. I had been unable to get some balance in my perspective on my problems. We decided that I needed to address a pile of unresolved anger regarding my employer and a previous accident, and some anger with my husband over household chores. He had been feeling that I'd just given up, and he was resentful about having to do so much housework on top of his job when he thought I could still do some of it. I also decided, at her suggestion, to practice some stress-reducing exercises, which have helped a lot. I was way more stressed than I knew. I probably hadn't taken a really deep breath in I don't know how long.

Also at her suggestion, I found and joined a support group for people who have chronic pain problems. I can't describe how much this helped me. I was nervous about going at first. I felt pretty self-conscious, but everyone there was very welcoming. Here was a group of people, different ages with different pain problems, who really understood what I was going through. Even after the first meeting, I felt better—not physically, but emotionally. Since then, I've gotten some great ideas about dealing with my situation. And I have gotten over feeling sorry for myself so much now.

Am I pain free now? No, but I do feel that I'm more in control of things now. I still have some bad days, but overall, I'm a lot more positive about everything. In fact, my husband and I are actually planning a vacation together, the first in a long time.

Polarized thinking and a feeling of hopelessness, mixed with a fair amount of anger and frustration: that recipe had kept

Paula from taking any steps to make her life better despite her pain. With the help of her doctor and her support group, however, Paula was able to look at her situation in a new way. She was able to identify the issues that were holding her back and then address them. Simply discovering that she wasn't helpless, that she could take control and work to make her situation better, made an enormous difference.

Beyond Support: Have a Plan

It's important to recognize the potential challenges that lie ahead and then to develop a plan to address them. The psychological aspects are especially important for any person trying to get over these hurdles.

We have emphasized the value of support groups, but it's also important to have some trusted and objective person to talk with, be it your doctor, a sponsor, a loved one, or maybe a friend who's in recovery. You need someone to whom you can say: "Here's my plan going into this situation. We both agreed that it's okay, but when I'm in the heat of the moment, and I've got to decide whether I'm going to take another pain pill or try a warm compress, I want to be able to call you and talk to you about it."

If your support person says, "No, it doesn't sound like you're sticking to the plan," you need to be able to listen to him or her.

Jake, the man you read about in the introduction, is a good example of a person taking a proactive approach. He explored and tried a variety of therapies for his knee pain, including massage therapy and yoga. Once he and his doctors agreed that the best option was surgery, they met to lay out a plan for dealing with postoperative pain, a plan that included some opioids and a number of complementary therapies. Jake also talked about his upcoming surgery with his sponsor and his recovery meeting. He told everyone why he needed surgery, laid out his plans for controlling pain, and went back to his meeting as soon as he could to let everyone know how things were going. Jake's surgeon and family doctor were also pleased with the results. They, too, were concerned about his recovery because they knew of people who had relapsed in similar situations, and they were more than happy to work with him on a pain control plan that would minimize the risk of relapse.

Ask Not What Your Doctor Can Do for You . . .

Most people are familiar with the late President John F. Kennedy's words, "Ask not what your country can do for you; ask what you can do for your country." We have paraphrased this concept: "Ask not what your doctor can do for you; ask what you can do for your doctor—and for yourself, with your doctor's help." Here we are emphasizing the patient's side of the relationship. How can you take responsibility for your health? What does your doctor expect from you? If you are in recovery, the self-knowledge you gained in that process should help you decide which tools will work for you, given your own strengths and weaknesses. As a result, you could be in a much better position than the average person to formulate your strategy. Then, ask your doctor to come on board. This is a much better plan than taking a passive approach that leaves everything in the hands of your doctor, who may pick techniques or approaches that aren't best suited to you. In addition, you'll have much more ownership in a plan you contributed to than in one someone else created. Yours will likely be well thought through.

Talk about your plan and the whole process of addressing your pain with your sponsor and the other support people in your life. By doing so, you'll come up with better ideas than you would have on your own. Equally important, if you are in recovery, you know that acting alone and being secretive is always a warning signal. Invite other people into the process.

Documenting Your Results

Keeping a record of your progress and setbacks, medications and physical therapies, is important for both you and your doctor. A daily pain management journal will help you and your doctor determine the therapies that help most, and you'll have a reasonably objective means of tracking your progress over time, rather than relying on nebulous impressions. Generally, people tend to remember what works and forget what doesn't, but with a journal, you'll have an easy, effective means of measuring your progress over weeks or months.

Keeping a journal can serve another important purpose for people in recovery from addiction to alcohol or other drugs. If you are faced with the decision about whether to use opioids, having an objective record that includes the treatments you've tried, their results, and the decisions you've made about them is extremely valuable. At that point, you would know that you'd done everything you could to alleviate your pain and that it now might make sense to seriously consider using an opioid—a difficult decision that can be fraught with worry and guilt. For tips on starting and keeping your own journal, refer to appendix C.

What's more, an objective record would be an enormous help for a physician who might prescribe opioids for you. You could say, for example, "Look, I've tried a dozen different ways to manage the pain and I've spelled out how I've responded to them, how long I tried them, at what dose and frequency, and here's the outcome: my level of pain and my level of activity." This kind of documentation would give your doctor solid facts about the treatments you've tried and their results, showing how hard you've worked to solve your pain problem. It could also reveal treatments or medications you had perhaps overlooked that might be effective. With this kind of information at hand, a doctor could recommend the best and most appropriate treatments for you.

CHAPTER 7

Pain Control and Relapse

The Medical Debate

Today, medical practice has determined that pain must be considered when evaluating the basic condition of a person seeking medical care. In fact, pain has been termed the fifth vital sign, along with body temperature, pulse, blood pressure, and respiration.

Exactly how aggressively should doctors treat pain? Before addressing this question, it's important to see how our attitudes as a society toward pain have changed over time. Not so long ago, we thought that pain was something we just had to endure. We regarded complaining or looking for relief as a sign of weakness. Consider how many young boys were told, when they were hurt and sobbing, to be quiet because "big boys don't cry."

Nevertheless, a strong debate still continues over this very question in the United States, and it's framed along these lines. On the one hand are people who passionately believe that pain should be treated aggressively, that unnecessary suffering is wrong, and that all patients should be assessed for pain when they come into the hospital. They maintain that morphine and its derivatives, the opioids, are proven effective for control of pain and that they really are quite safe when used correctly. As long as opioids are given in appropriate doses under close medical supervision, patients will not have damage to their stomach, liver, or kidneys (opioids are in fact safer in this regard than NSAIDs or acetaminophen). Nor are breathing problems likely with opioid use, except in the case of overdose or in combination with other sedating medications. These proponents also feel that the risk of addiction is very low.

The counterargument focuses primarily on the addictive potential of opioids. The opioid medications clearly relieve pain very effectively, but they also have addictive properties— and herein lies the crux of the debate that is ongoing in the United States.

Opponents believe that drug abuse is rampant in certain populations in the United States. They argue that making opioids more readily available or prescribing them more often will make this problem worse and create more addicts who won't be productive members of society. Certainly, there have been inappropriate prescriptions of these drugs, and pharmacists and physicians have been prosecuted for criminal offenses for knowingly entering into illicit agreements and selling prescriptions of these drugs. The abuse of OxyContin, for example, is well documented.

Although opioid medications, such as morphine and codeine, can be very addictive, when they are taken for pain as directed by a physician, the risk of addiction *for the average person* seems to be small (although little research exists in this area). This is definitely *not* the case, however, for people in recovery from alcoholism or other substance abuse. These individuals must be extremely careful about using any opioid (see chapter 8).

Proponents of these two views are continually going head to head, and physicians are often caught in the middle. The treatment of pain is getting a lot of attention today because there's a sense that physicians have not treated pain adequately, thus allowing needless suffering. At the same time, there has been a fear on the part of many physicians that if they prescribe opioids too often for pain, they will be called before the medical board. This fear is, in fact, warranted, because physicians in several states have gotten into trouble for *appropriately* prescribing opioids. They want to do what is medically best for their patients, but they don't want to be accused by the government of overprescribing opioids.

Patients are likewise caught in the middle. If people have pain, of course they want to be helped. They may go to their doctor legitimately seeking relief, and they want to have all the options available to them. Neither they nor their doctor wants to create a situation in which someone becomes addicted. There is no easy answer, however, simply because of the nature of opioids. They have a positive side and a dark side as well.

Recovering addicts, especially former opioid addicts, are often undertreated for their pain. When physicians know of the addiction, they may appropriately hesitate to give potentially addictive medications. What's more, because of their addiction history, these individuals may need higher doses than the average person because they have developed a residual tolerance to opioids.

A brief look at some facts scientists have discovered over the years can help us understand these issues. When researchers first purified morphine from opium, they quickly saw its positive and negative effects. In recent years, we have discovered that the human body has molecules it uses every day for modulating pain, molecules that look a lot like morphine. These are the endogenous opioids called enkephalins and endorphins. Morphine is a plant-derived molecule that just happens to look and *act* a lot like what the body is already using.

Once researchers discovered this, they began trying to synthesize a molecule that would specifically fit in the pain relief keyhole without causing addiction or other side effects like nausea, vomiting, sedation, or respiratory depression. Unfortunately, despite a huge effort, they have not found this magic key, although they continue to try. In recent years, some new drugs initially seemed to be "the one," only to be found wrong. History has repeated itself so many times, however, that it's wiser to accept the opioids for what they are and use them carefully.

Generally speaking, from your health care provider's perspective, a history of substance abuse raises a large red flag when he or she is considering prescribing opioids, particularly for a long-term pain problem. However, this is *not* to say that it's impossible for a person with a history of alcohol or other drug abuse or dependency to use opioids safely. Jake's story in the introduction illustrates this point.

This book provides information to help people with addiction histories properly treat pain while reducing relapse risk as much as possible. Of course, opioids always entail some degree of risk because of their inherent addictive properties. But that risk must be weighed against the hazards of untreated pain. Moreover, that risk can be minimized by using opioids within a structured plan and support system. In this chapter, you'll learn more about how these risks can be wisely balanced.

Effects of Opioids

When treating acute pain, physicians attempt to relieve pain immediately, and that's commonly done with medications. Unrelieved pain has many negative effects, including a slower recovery from surgery and lowered immunity to disease. For people with chronic pain, treatment goals are more complicated. Pain relief is important, certainly, but so is helping patients continue to function at work and to enjoy social and leisure activities.

These two goals—pain relief and improved function— sometimes conflict with one another. Opioids are effective pain relievers when taken in small amounts for a short time. They generally cause only minor side effects. But when they are taken in larger doses for several weeks or months, the side effects can become limiting, including nausea, vomiting, sleepiness, loss of appetite, and constipation. More sinister is the possible effect of opioids on drive and motivation, which may impair functional recovery.

Opioids can also produce what is described as "rebound pain." The effect of some opioids, for example, lasts only a few hours. Pain can return as these short-acting medications wear off or when they are withdrawn from a patient's treatment. Interestingly, opioids can also cause changes in people's nervous systems that actually heighten their perception of pain and make them feel more uncomfortable. This is called *opioid-induced hyperalgesia*. This phenomenon is analogous to tolerance. In this case, however, not only do the pain pathways from the nociceptive source become tolerant to opioids, but the body's own endogenous opiate receptors also become tolerant. As a result, you lose some of your own ability to regulate your pain. This is a new discovery, and while scientists don't know exactly how significant this phenomenon is in humans, it might explain why some people just don't do well using opioids in the long term.

Chronic exposure to opioids can also decrease the level of testosterone and adversely affect a person's sex drive. Because opioids have so many effects, both positive and negative, and because the medical community has some concern about their lack of effectiveness for treating some types of pain, some doctors restrict the use of opioids when treating chronic pain. They may also be uneasy about the possible long-term side effects, which can interfere with rehabilitation and lead to more doctor visits and hospital stays.

Opioids: Pain Relief versus an Addictive High

To understand the dual effects of opioids, think of a person who has neither a problem with pain nor any history of substance abuse. We'll call this state "normal." Let's say that such a patient has had surgery and is just awakening from anesthesia in severe pain. A nurse comes into the room and gives morphine; soon the pain is gone and the patient feels relatively "normal" again.

Used in this way, morphine brings people back to the "normal" state of being pain free. They do not, however, feel any euphoria from the medicine; rather, they feel only relief from pain. Their body's reward circuits are not triggered, and they have no lingering desire to have the drug again, except perhaps to relieve their pain. This is the goal of treatment with morphine and other opioids: relieve pain without stimulating the reward centers of the brain that are associated with addictive behavior.

Let's say, however, that your experience with opioids is not directed by a doctor, and you're not starting out in pain. If you take opioids, you *will* stimulate your brain's reward center and move into a state of euphoria. This is how addiction begins, especially in individuals with a genetic predisposition to addiction. Thus the same opioid can have two very different effects depending on the dose and the circumstances under which it's used. This is also the reason that if a doctor gives an opioid to a person who takes it strictly as directed for the relief of pain, in general there's little risk that he or she will become addicted, while the same drug and dose given to a different person under other circumstances could precipitate a fall into addiction.

Factors Working against People in Recovery

People with a history of substance abuse know that they may be putting themselves at risk by using opioids. Given this prior struggle with addictive behavior, they are at greater risk for relapse by using such drugs, even in a monitored health care setting. They and their health care providers need to be concerned about some important factors when considering the use of opioids, including their genetic predisposition for the addictive consequence and their memory, conscious or not, of the high they felt when taking drugs.

We know that withdrawal and abstinence can be achieved

in a relatively short period of time, but the memory of the addictive experience is powerful and can last a lifetime. A recovering addict may have cravings from time to time that a person with no prior drug-using behavior would not have. Someone in recovery from opioid addiction, for example, may find that while the correct dose of an intravenous pain medication does not trigger any high, simply watching a needle being used to deliver drugs could easily trigger powerful memories of drug use and strong cravings for drugs again.

Research with alcohol use seems to indicate that there is a biological reason for this behavior. If the brain cells are regularly "bathed" in alcohol, the protein structure of the cell will actually change over time so that eventually it will function at its peak only in the presence of the alcohol. We think now that after a period of sobriety, the cells will eventually return to a normal state again, in which peak functioning takes place only *without* the presence of alcohol. Somehow a cellular memory of the addicted state remains, however, and the reintroduction of alcohol can cause a rapid return of brain cell response to the addictive state.

Cross-addiction might also be facilitated by this kind of brain response. We know that it's not uncommon for an addicted person to stop using his or her drug of choice, such as alcohol, only to turn to another substance, which quickly becomes the new addiction. Some kind of cellular memory might also be at work in this situation.

We also know that cravings and even relapse can be triggered simply by people, places, and paraphernalia connected to recovering addicts' using behaviors. Examples include just being in the same area where they used to buy drugs, watching a scene in a movie that shows use of a drug they used, seeing a bong in a store window, or having a nurse tie off an arm for a blood test.

Understanding that such situations could trigger cravings was an important discovery. A person in recovery may have licked his or her actual drug dependency and be years away from withdrawal but still feel the psychological effects, even if unintended, from an appropriately prescribed opioid painkiller solely because of memories, feelings, and emotions the drug brings up. Given that this is possible, reexperiencing even a bit of euphoria associated with pain treatment could be extremely risky for people in recovery, regardless of the addictive chemicals they formerly used.

Risk Factors for Addiction

A number of factors can play a role in creating a situation in which people become addicted to a particular drug.

Availability. Whether a drug is licit or illicit, its availability directly affects how much it's used. Opioid addiction is limited among the general U.S. population because most people have little access to opioids unless they're having surgery or otherwise dealing with severe pain. Conversely, in the course of their work, anesthesiologists have fairly easy access to most opioids; they also have an increased risk, as a group, of addiction to this class of drugs.

Cost. Social science and medical science research clearly demonstrates that as the cost of cigarettes and alcohol rises, fewer people use these two addictive substances. Research has also shown, for example, that when the price of OxyContin rises, people addicted to it seek out heroin as a substitute.

Speed of delivery. The speed at which a drug affects the brain seems to be directly correlated to its addictive potential. There are three ways, for example, to use cocaine: snorting, injecting, and smoking. Snorting cocaine is the slowest "delivery" method. When cocaine is snorted, it has first to pass through the lining of the nose, then go into the bloodstream, before it can move on to the brain. Injecting the drug works more quickly, but the quickest way to get cocaine to the brain is to smoke it. This is one reason why crack cocaine is so addictive. Studies have shown that people who smoke cocaine have a greater chance of becoming addicted than do people who snort it. Similarly, in the case of two prescription drugs, the risk of addiction to alprazolam (Xanax) may be greater than with its related predecessor diazepam (Valium), because alprazolam is faster acting and therefore more reinforcing.

Cultural milieu. How one's culture views the use of a drug plays an important role in addiction levels. For example, the population of Utah has a much lower rate of alcohol addiction than does the rest of the country, in large part because its population is dominated by Mormons, whose religion forbids its use. In the Jewish culture, the use of alcohol is quite ritualistic and intoxication is frowned upon. Relatively low rates of alcoholism are related to these cultural factors.

Levels of peer pressure and social acceptance are additional factors that influence the use of a drug. Teenagers living in a community in which many of their peers drink alcohol and smoke marijuana are much more likely to use them than are youngsters living in an area where use and acceptability are more limited. For many years, a kind of taboo against heroin use existed among more affluent Americans. In recent years, however, that bias dissipated for some reason, and now its use has risen dramatically among affluent teens.

Environmental factors and genetics. A number of factors in this category seem to increase greatly the incidence of addiction, including a family history of addiction, mental illness, and significant family dysfunction such as violence, abuse, neglect, and sexual molestation. Researchers describe genetic factors as composing 55 percent of the risk of addiction; therefore environmental factors compose 45 percent.

Medical staff and patients should take these factors into account and work hard to control them as best they can with people who are going to use opioids for pain control. Access to the drugs, for example, is limited to the prescribed amount. Cost can play a role, because insurance plans will only pay for prescribed medications. In addition, doctors can control the speed at which an opioid reaches the brain: the fentanyl patch, for example, delivers pain medication much more slowly than an injection does. Finally, the cultural milieu of the medical world certainly differs significantly from the street milieu. The careful process of determining the kind of pain medication a patient can take and how it will be delivered takes into account environmental and genetic factors as well as any previous drug history.

Emotional and Psychological Pain and Addiction

Jason had a history of significant childhood trauma for which he'd never received help. He struggled in school, became addicted to alcohol and marijuana, and finally dropped out of school in eleventh grade.

At the age of nineteen, Jason managed to get through an out-patient treatment program and stopped using both drugs. Four years later, he was working on an assembly line in a small tool-and-die shop making little more than minimum wage. With few viable job skills and no education, this was the best he could do, and he wasn't really earning enough to support himself. He had the ever-present stress of wondering how he was going to get by as he juggled rent, utilities, food, and other expenses.

One day at work, Jason missed a rung going down a ladder and injured his knee badly enough to require surgery. The post-surgery pain medications, he suddenly realized, relieved not only the pain in his knee, but also the mental pain burdening him from a life of struggle and frustration and emotional stress. Jason began thinking about how he could manage to continue taking these drugs after his release from the hospital.

What happened to Jason is the psychological parallel to physically moving from a state of pain to one in which the pain is no longer present. While no euphoric feelings are produced by pain medications in Jason's case, to feel relief from years of psychological pain could easily propel an individual into overuse and even addiction if that pain is not addressed in any other way.

When we talk about pain, we tend to use many of the same words to describe physical pain, such as a burn or a sprain, and psychological pain. For example, it's not unusual to hear the emotional pain of a divorce or the death of a loved one described as an ache or pain that is incapacitating, crippling, devastating, or paralyzing.

We have already described, in chapter 1, how physical pain has an emotional component, and the medications we use provide relief, to some extent, for both aspects. In a very real sense, then, these parallel descriptions of psychic and bodily pain found in our language may have a basis in the fact that they are "felt" in the same area of the brain. The link between relieving a hurt and feeling good, whether we do it pharmacologically or by meeting a basic physical or emotional need, may put certain individuals who are also suffering from unrecognized or unresolved psychological pain at risk. Taking a medication for a physical pain might also bring relief from emotional pain, and a powerful sense of relief could lead them into addictive behavior.

As a society, we don't address chronic physical pain and chronic emotional pain to the same degree. For example, it would be difficult to find people who have endured tremendous physical pain without trying to relieve it. Psychological trauma, however, is often repressed and left unrecognized and untreated for years. Note, for instance, that virtually all physical illnesses are covered by medical insurance plans, while few plans will cover psychological counseling or extensive treatment for mental illnesses in the same manner. Admitting to emotional problems, depression, or mental illness is still seen as a sign of weakness.

In the addiction field, it's not unusual for people in recovery to talk about their chemical use in terms of "self-medicating." In other words, they feel that they were, either consciously or unconsciously, using alcohol or other drugs to ease emotional pain. Even if this action was on an unconscious level, they did feel some relief, albeit eventually with very negative consequences.

Pain is uncomfortable, and humans have an innate drive to relieve pain, whether physical or emotional, even if that means trying anything that promises to help, addictive substances included. To some extent, this "hurt" we discussed, whether it's brought on through psychological trauma or physical pain, may be the same experience. At the very least, we know that many of the medications that relieve one type of pain will relieve the other, too.

It is precisely because pain-relieving medicines affect both kinds of pain that it is so important for people with psychological, emotional pain to address these behavioral and emotional issues before they begin using opioids or other medications that can be addictive. If patients can be successful in at least identifying these issues, then they can more safely consider an opioid for pain. This awareness will help them recognize the drug's effect on both pain and behavior, as well as its effect on their mood or psychic distress.

Admittedly, this can be a tough knot to untie. This is, again, an important reason why opioids should be used with caution and why people in recovery should take particular care. Someone else must control when and how they take these medications to protect them from inadvertently falling into an addictive pattern. If, for example, they take an opioid that for whatever reason is "rewarding" because it relieved either psychic pain or physical pain or because it produced some feelings of euphoria, that behavioral connection between feeling pain relief and deciding to take the pills needs to be avoided or taken out of their control. Someone else—medical staff, a family member, or a sponsor—must have the responsibility to decide when the medication should be taken and at what dose. (See appendix D, "Guidelines for Safely Taking Addictive Medications.")

This discussion of risk factors associated with the potential for relapse or addiction should help you recognize the need for an organized, careful, and thoughtful approach to the treatment of pain while in recovery. Assessing your risks with the help of your health care professionals can provide valuable information as you make these difficult decisions. The added risk of being in recovery does not mean that one should always avoid opioids. Instead, it can provide the motivation for exploring options and using the tools described in this book to minimize risk.

CHAPTER 8

Considering Opioids for Pain

Despite the debate over their use, opioids can be a key part of a treatment plan for people in recovery, particularly to address acute pain for a brief period. Such was the case for Jake, the patient described in the introduction, who was prescribed oxycodone with acetaminophen (Percocet) for pain following knee surgery. However, for chronic pain, opioids present more challenges, both for you and for your medical team. In this chapter, we'll examine the range of concerns involved and appropriate ways to address them.

In the 1800s, salesmen with patent medicine wagons roamed throughout the United States selling opium elixirs and leaving a goodly number of addicts in their wake. The pendulum has swung back and forth on the question of opioids for a century, alternating between liberal use without acknowledging the danger to periods of very restrictive use, the most recent of which occurred in the 1970s. Some in the medical community at that time were so restrictive with morphine that they were reticent to prescribe opioids for people dying of cancer because of concerns about addiction.

Both camps have viable arguments, and we have valuable lessons to learn from this history. Doctors have been inextricably linked to society's pendulum swings. These trends are not just historical; there are also geographical trends and medical specialty trends—oncologists versus internists, for example—that differ on this issue. In this book we take a prudent approach that attempts to balance the dilemma.

Relieving chronic pain can be difficult to achieve at times. Anybody can have problems as a result of poorly monitored and inappropriate use of opioids. Treatment centers do see patients, for example, who've been prescribed opioids for pain and who, as a result of poor monitoring, were no longer working or doing much at all besides lying listlessly and watching TV. This may be pain relief, but it's at an unacceptable cost.

Some of the blame for such situations lies at the feet of the medical community. Although there has been some improvement, medical students still receive insufficient training in the areas of both chemical dependency and pain control. Making matters worse, our current medical system focuses on physician "productivity," which means that doctors are expected to see many patients each day. This can interfere with the doctor's time to address the issue of opioid pain control for someone in recovery.

To deal with pain as we have suggested, and especially chronic pain, takes time. At a minimum, a thirty- to sixty-minute initial conversation is needed with the patient, other caregivers, and family members. More time is needed if the patient has had problems with alcohol or other drugs in the past. That's a lot of time in today's health care environment. It is quicker and simpler for a doctor to write a prescription for a pain medication and send patients on their way.

Conversely, too many patients are unwilling to make the effort needed to explore rehabilitative and psychological therapies that could give them pain control. Instead, they seek out a quick fix and doctors who they know will simply prescribe a pain medication.

Combine these two factors, and it's easy to understand why some doctors don't pursue the most appropriate course of action as often as they should. In this chapter, however, you will find the information you need to avoid such situations and to receive the care you want and need.

Using Opioids for Acute Pain

In general, we recommend that people who have had a previous history of abuse or addiction to alcohol or other drugs, particularly with opioids, should avoid using opioids if at all possible. As we noted in previous chapters, pain treatment can be approached with a number of medicines and modalities, and all appropriate approaches should be considered before making a decision to use opioids.

That being said, it's nevertheless essential to understand that opioids can be safe and very effective, even for people in recovery. A history of substance abuse obviously creates a special situation, but opioids should not be ruled out simply because of a problem with addiction in general or opioid addiction in particular. No one, including people with a history of substance abuse, should have to suffer from pain that would respond to treatment.

Using opioids for acute or short-term pain, such as after surgery or a dental procedure, potentially presents less of a problem than using them to control chronic pain. We've previously noted that it's rare, for example, for a person using morphine or another opioid for postoperative pain to experience relapse or euphoria. In such cases, these medicines actually have a sedating effect. Nor do *most* people become addicted to opioids when they are used in such situations, even though many people fear such an outcome.

Many people in recovery have used opioids after surgery or for other situations in which they were in extreme pain requiring opioid medication for a brief period. Brad is one of them.

I am a pharmacist working at a chemical dependency treatment center. Three years ago, I needed surgery on my spine. I knew that my postsurgical pain would be severe and that morphine would be the best drug to deal with that pain. I'd been clean and sober for fifteen years after having been addicted to cocaine for three years. I was nervous about using an opioid for pain control, but after talking over my concerns with two pain specialists and with my center's medical director, we came to the conclusion that in this circumstance, with close supervision, I could use morphine. After the surgery, I was using a morphine pump, and I didn't feel any of the high I used to feel with cocaine. The only thing my doctors noticed that might have been related to my addiction was that I seemed to need a little higher dose to control my pain than most people need. They thought that since I'd been addicted in the past, perhaps I still carried some kind of tolerance to these drugs.

Letting people with a history of addiction decide on their own about medication use would put them in a precarious position. However, legitimately using the medication for only a short period with strict supervision and controls—such as scheduled dosing to prevent the individual from making dosage decisions—can be done without undue risk of triggering relapse. In these situations, some recovering people even choose to bring an AA or NA meeting into their home after surgery for support. They also make a point of talking with their sponsors and other close friends in recovery about their use of opioid medications.

Guidelines for Using Opioids to Treat Acute Pain

The following set of precautionary steps and specific guidelines are designed to help people in recovery safely use opioids for short-term pain.

- Approach the use of opioids carefully and with the full disclosure of all past alcohol or other drug use.
- When thinking about opioids, consider your full range of options. Ask about the possibility of combining them with simple analgesics and physical modalities for maximum pain relief.
- The dose and frequency should be prescribed and scheduled by a doctor. No one with a history of substance abuse should be prescribed a potentially addictive drug on a "take as needed" basis. Especially under the pressure—or the "excuse"—of pain, a patient could too easily decide "It felt okay when I took two for pain, so maybe three or four would help even more." Too high a dose could push the drug's effect past mere pain relief into the abuse or euphoria-producing range. And there begins the slippery, and steep, slope into relapse and addiction.
- You and your doctor should make a commitment that you will use these medications for the shortest

possible period of time, after which you will turn
to nonaddictive medicines and/or nonpharmacological methods, discussed earlier in this book.

- If pain control needs to be addressed after a dental
  or surgical procedure, involve the whole health
  care team in a discussion in which you address all
  the concerns and possible outcomes. Make a list of
  issues to discuss with your doctor and create a plan
  that addresses the kind of anesthetic that will be
  used, a detailed plan for managing the pain afterward, and a backup plan in case "plan A" is not
  effective.

- Consider a consultation with an addiction medicine
  specialist.

With a well-thought-out plan in place ahead of time, you
should be able to manage pain effectively and recover suc-
cessfully with no addiction-related problems. (Side effects of
medications, such as nausea, constipation, or itching can still
occur.)

The experiences of Jake and Kathleen, described in the introduction, show both sides of this issue. Kathleen didn't discuss her concerns about relapse with anyone, not her dentist,
her sponsor, or her Twelve Step meeting. She clearly did not
have a plan to address her pain if it became too much for her
to bear. Had she spoken with her dentist about her concerns
and taken the other steps we've described, she could have
avoided the unfortunate relapse that eventually resulted.

Jake took the opposite approach. Before his surgery, he
arranged a meeting with his family doctor and the orthopedist who would do his surgery to discuss pain control both

right after surgery and during his rehabilitation. The plan the three of them set up included an "opioid agreement" (see appendix D) that carefully spelled out how he would use opioid medicines after surgery to control his pain, how his use would be monitored to ensure that he wouldn't trigger a relapse, and when he would switch to nonopioid medications and complementary therapies for his pain. In addition, Jake was also open about his surgery and medication plan with his sponsor and members of his AA meeting. The promise of care and support from these people helped him feel more at ease about the surgery and more confident that he could get through the process and manage any problems.

Using Opioids for Chronic Pain

At this point, we have accepted that a person with a history of addiction should, by taking the precautionary steps we've laid out, be able to take a minimal amount of opioid medication for the minimum amount of time needed to recover from postsurgical or other acute, short-term pain.

Until now, however, we have avoided the toughest problem: What about the recovering person who is suffering with chronic pain and for whom "everything" has already been done? Should such a person be a candidate for taking opioids for chronic pain? Is it possible for a person in recovery to control the use of opioids for a long period of time?

These questions are regularly being debated throughout the country in both the medical and addiction treatment fields. Some pain experts take a stance that says all those in recovery should be treated as though they do not have this risk of relapse and addiction. On the issue's opposite side are some addiction professionals who recommend that *no one* in recovery should be prescribed opioids. We believe that each of these views is too extreme. While we do have strong reservations about prescribing opioids for chronic pain, we nevertheless remain open to considering them in special circumstances.

Criteria for Using Opioids to Treat Chronic Pain

If you and your doctor are seriously considering the use of opioids for chronic pain and if you have a history of substance abuse, several stringent criteria must be met before such use can begin—criteria, frankly, that are necessarily quite difficult to meet. They include the following:

- Researching and trying nonopioid pharmacological and nonpharmacological medical treatments, including complementary treatment programs such as acupuncture, therapeutic massage, biofeedback, or movement therapies. (See chapter 5 for more on complementary medicine.)
- Using psychological or cognitive behavioral therapies that address pain and are designed principally to improve function, *regardless of pain,* such as stress-relief techniques, lifestyle changes, and relaxation techniques. (See chapter 6 for a discussion of psychological approaches to pain.)
- Working in close collaboration with a health care team who will monitor you closely, perhaps more closely than is comfortable for you.
- Measuring your success by your functionality, not

just your pain relief. Medical staff and other support persons will monitor your medication use and pain relief, but other behavior-related checks and balances must also be in place. Pay attention to your ability to function and your activity levels. You and your health care team should note how these compare to your "normal" standards. Are you getting to work and performing acceptably? Are you doing household chores? Maintaining relationships? Becoming more, rather than less, active? Or is your behavior becoming aberrant? If behavioral problems appear in such areas, serious questions should be raised about the medications' effectiveness, and also about their possible contribution to these problems.

Choosing a Doctor and Medical Facility

Ideally, you should have one primary care doctor who can coordinate all your care and medications. If you are seeing a number of doctors and aren't careful about communicating with them, you may find yourself in a situation in which none of your doctors has a complete view of your care.

If you have a chronic pain problem that your primary care doctor is not able to treat, or if he or she is comfortable only with a limited number of pain drugs, you should consider asking for a referral to a pain specialist, especially if you are in recovery. If you do, however, be sure to stay in touch with your primary care doctor and keep him or her abreast of your treatment progress.

How to Find a Pain Doctor

Let your primary care doctor give you some suggestions. Possibilities would include a specialist in pain medicine, physical medicine and rehabilitation, or neurology. While most physician specialists have expertise in treating particular diseases or organ systems, pain specialists are different. They are experts in understanding and managing a complex and variable symptom—pain—as a condition in its own right, no matter its cause. Pain specialists often work at facilities called pain centers or pain clinics.

Some pain clinics focus primarily on one mode of pain treatment, such as steroid injections to reduce inflammation. Others specialize in treating one particular type of pain, such as headaches or back pain. Pain centers affiliated with universities or medical schools typically provide more comprehensive services with a broader variety of specialists and treatment methods.

Each type of pain clinic has particular advantages and disadvantages. A comprehensive program, for example, can offer more variety, which in turn will give you a greater chance of finding an effective treatment. Such comprehensive centers are less common than specialty clinics, and as a result, you may have to travel farther to find one.

Clinics that focus on one method of treatment are generally easier to find, less expensive, and less time-consuming. But if a clinic's particular type of treatment doesn't work for you, it may be difficult to receive other kinds of treatment there, and as a result, you may not get the treatment that's best for you.

Find the Cause First

If you don't know, or aren't sure of, the cause of your pain, your first step should be to find the cause. A correct diagnosis makes it easier to choose effective treatments. You also want to make certain that your pain is not a sign of some underlying disease, such as an infection or cancer.

Your primary care doctor may refer you to several specialists or even to a pain center or clinic if the cause of your pain is unclear. You may need to undergo a number of diagnostic tests and try a variety of treatments. Be sure your doctors clearly explain the risks and benefits of any treatment they suggest. Equally important, they need to know about your addiction history.

Find the Experts

To find a reputable pain program that fits your needs, talk with your doctor. Some programs require a letter of referral from your primary care doctor and a copy of your medical records.

If you live near a medical school, find out if it has a pain center or clinic. If you're attending a support group for your pain or illness, talk to members of the group who have been to a pain facility and listen to their opinions on that program.

Finally, consider contacting the National Pain Foundation or the American Pain Foundation to find out about pain resources in your area. More information can be found on their Web sites: for the National Pain Foundation, see www.painconnection.org; for the American Pain Foundation, see www.painfoundation.org.

Choosing a Clinic or Medical Center

Facilities and personnel vary in their qualifications and focus, so consider these factors when evaluating your options.

What are the goals? Is the program focused strictly on relieving patients' pain, or does it include services to help determine the cause of pain or personal problems that may be associated with pain? In other words, does it focus *both* on your pain and on your lifestyle, behavior, and activities—or just on your pain?

What methods does it advocate? Be particularly careful in evaluating programs that routinely include surgery, that rely on unproven therapies, or that advocate only the long-term use of potentially addictive drugs, such as opioids.

Are the program and staff accredited or certified? Pain physicians can be certified by specialty boards, including the American Board of Anesthesiology, the American Board of Pain Medicine, the American Board of Physical Medicine and Rehabilitation, and the American Board of Neurology and Psychiatry. Certification also helps ensure that the program meets the basic requirements for appropriate medical care.

Does it have a good success rate? Ask to see the statistics on the program's long-term success rate. Of course, no program can promise a 100 percent success rate. That rate also depends on the age and composition of the population treated.

Does it include follow-up services? If you need additional care once you've completed your treatment, there should be a person at the center whom you can contact. Avoid programs that offer no follow-up care.

What about its cost? Cost is always a consideration, so be sure that you know approximately how much the treatment will cost before you begin. Check with your insurance company to see what expenses will be covered. Some insurance companies cover treatment provided by comprehensive pain programs while others do not. Coverage of different types of treatment and services associated with specialized pain facilities also varies among insurance policies. You may have to write to your insurance company to get approval in advance for specialized pain treatments.

Remember Your Role in Your Health Care

As we have noted, your participation in a program at a pain center or clinic is similar to many efforts in life. What you receive from the experience is directly related to the effort you put into it. If you have little faith in your ability to learn new skills and low expectations about your recovery prospects, it's likely that the program won't give you the results you desire. But if you have a positive attitude and realistic expectations, you'll gain control over some aspects of your pain and learn how to get maximum benefit from treatment. Knowledge and control will, in turn, give you the confidence to deal effectively with your pain. Attitude, commitment, and expectations matter regardless of the cause of the pain.

Talk to Your Doctor about Your Addiction History

If you've reached a point where you believe that you need to try an opioid to achieve the level of pain relief you want, you must have a discussion with your doctor, one in which you are completely open about your medical and addiction history. You must clearly state your willingness and commitment to take whatever steps are needed for you to use opioids safely. Your doctor needs to know about your addiction history in order to do all he or she can to help you achieve adequate pain relief while minimizing as much as possible the risk of relapse.

It's important to recognize, however, that many in the medical community are inadequately trained to handle such situations. In medical school, most students receive only one or two lectures about pain and substance abuse. In day-to-day practice, it's easier and more commonplace for general surgeons and internists to ignore the problem. In our current medical care system, it's still easier for a doctor to give a prescription than to sit down and really talk with and teach a patient.

If you're going to have surgery done by a general surgeon and you say to him or her, "Look, I'm in recovery from drug abuse and I'm worried about pain medications triggering a relapse, so I need to be careful about how much I take," it would not be surprising for the surgeon to refuse to prescribe any opioid medication for you, or provide a low dose that is likely to be safe but is inadequate for pain relief.

Patients would instead do well to take the initiative and come up with a plan ahead of time. If you tell your doctor, for example, "I'm a recovering addict, so I have certain risk factors that might make you reluctant to work with me. I know it's going to take more effort on both our parts to address this problem, but I'm willing to do whatever it takes to make this work," your doctor should be more receptive to working with you. You might also tell your doctor that you read this book and that it provided you with guidelines on areas to cover. Tell the doctor that you've drawn up a plan, and then review it together. Your doctor would be able to look it over and quickly discern whether it's reasonable and whether he or she could support it.

Most physicians won't create that plan for you for two reasons: they have neither the time nor the training to do it. Such a plan needs to be individualized to the kind of tools each individual patient finds effective and knows how to use. On the other hand, most physicians and surgeons would be open to such a plan if you've been comprehensive and thoughtful, and they would certainly fill in the medical portions as needed. They could be highly motivated to do their part to really help you.

If, however, you come to a doctor or surgeon with a spotty drug use history, showing no investment in your own health and no ownership of your problems, it would be very easy for that doctor to ignore those problems or to encourage you to seek medical care elsewhere. Simply put, you'll have a better experience with a physician if you have "done your homework" and have made a commitment to be an active participant in your care.

Some years ago, Michele, sixty years old and sober from alcohol for twenty years, injured her back and ruptured a vertebral disk. For two years or so, however, her back pain was increasing. She'd tried some nonopioid pain medications, but they hadn't helped

enough, so her doctor prescribed hydrocodone with acetamino-
phen (Vicodin), which she'd used for eight months.

Michele never told her doctor about her alcoholism because
she felt that her use was so far in the past that it wasn't worth
mentioning. In addition, her doctor did not think to ask whether
she'd had any problems with chemical dependency, nor did he
talk much with her about the potential risk of addiction to hy-
drocodone. As a result, Michele wasn't concerned about taking
an opioid and didn't tell anybody about her use of pain medica-
tion. As tolerance to the drug increased, she began taking larger
doses, and slowly but surely, she began slipping into addiction.

Chronic pain initially led Michele to seek opioid medications,
but her isolation, her lack of involvement with other people, and
her failure to reveal her past problem with alcohol, combined
with chronic and worsening pain, led to her relapse.

Understand Your Doctor's Perspective about Opioids

We have previously discussed some of the fears doctors generally have when prescribing opioids, and those fears are com-
pounded when working with patients who have a history of
addiction. If you can understand, be sensitive to, and address
your doctor's concerns, you will increase the likelihood that
he or she will agree to pursue this line of treatment.

When approaching your doctor about using opioids for
control of chronic pain, consider the following steps.

Be honest and open from the very start. At your first appointment, you might begin by saying, "I need help with a pain
problem, I have a history of substance abuse, and I want to be
totally honest with you. You may be hesitant to work with me,

but I'll be completely open with you. I'm prepared to be committed to this process."

Bring trustworthy support people into the process at the beginning. Lying to yourself is a cardinal symptom of addiction, and lying to your doctor isn't too hard once you've lied to yourself. Only your friends and family know you well enough to catch the lies early; they may be able to spot a problem before you are aware of it. That's why you need their support. Involving a trusted group of people in your care gives support to a doctor who may be reluctant to trust a patient with an addiction history. Consider inviting your doctor to call your spouse or partner, your employer, or your AA or NA sponsor, for example, to check up on you. Or invite these people to some of your appointments. If trustworthy people are involved with your care, your doctor will gain confidence that he or she has an accurate picture of your situation.

Provide your medical records. Offer your doctor a copy of all your medical records. It's your right as a patient to withhold these records, but doing so would raise a significant red flag for your doctor. Be sure to list the other doctors you've seen and provide a complete medical history.

Promise exclusivity. Too often, people with chronic pain secretly use and get prescriptions from a number of different doctors. To address this concern, you might say, "If you agree to help me, I will agree to see only you. I'll promise not to go to other doctors and shop around for extra medications. And if I'm not happy with your care plan, I won't just drop you and go to the next doctor. I'll talk to you about my concerns and try to resolve them." With such reassurances, you'll demonstrate your commitment to the process and to your doctor.

Agree to use only one local pharmacy. Patients who abuse the system to acquire more medicine than they've been prescribed often try to fill the same prescription at multiple pharmacies. Tell your doctor that you'll also agree to use only one pharmacy for anything prescribed for you. Again, make it clear that you understand your doctor's concerns and that you're willing to take all these steps not only to reduce your risk of abusing the medication, but also to protect your physician from the scrutiny of peers, a medical association, or the U.S. Drug Enforcement Administration (DEA).

Reiterate your willingness to try other nonopioid and nonpharmacological approaches. Review your previous treatment history with your doctor. Let your doctor know that you're willing to first consider nonopioid and nonpharmacological approaches for your pain. You might say, "I've read *Pain-Free Living for Drug-Free People,* published by the Hazelden Foundation, so I've got some background on my problem. I understand your concerns. I don't really want to use opioids, and with luck, we'll find a way for me to avoid having to use them. But if opioids seem to be the only solution, I'd like you to consider them."

Be willing to commit to an agreement for safe use of addictive medications. (See "Using Opioids Safely," page 162, and appendix D.) Tell your doctor that you have a list of guidelines for safely taking addictive medications, and that you are willing to live by its stipulations. Bring a copy with you to your appointment and give it to your doctor. Your doctor may already have an equivalent agreement that is tailored to his or her practice. In this case, use what your doctor suggests.

Peter's Story

Peter, a prominent attorney, had been suffering with back pain for some years. He'd tried a variety of medicines and explored some complementary therapies, but still the pain remained. Eventually, he sought help at a well-known comprehensive pain clinic. After hearing his story and reviewing his medical records, Peter's doctor said, "Given everything you've done already, I'd suggest that it would make the most sense now to try an opioid medication for a while."

Peter was completely taken aback, and he responded that using an "addictive drug" would be a huge stigma in his profession. "If people knew that I was using narcotics, well, they just wouldn't understand," he replied. Peter and his doctor then had a long discussion about this problem. His doctor helped Peter look over all that he'd done to deal with his pain, and then addressed the concerns—and misconceptions— Peter had about opioid medications. In the end, Peter realized that he had indeed tried a variety of medications and therapies and that none of them had helped enough. He began taking an opioid as part of a comprehensive program and has continued to do so for a number of years without breaking his "agreement." Peter is functioning better now and continues to work nearly full time in his profession, although he still worries about potential problems with his colleagues if they should learn about his medications.

Using Opioids Safely

If you and your doctor conclude that it is appropriate for you to try taking an opioid for your pain, the first step the two of you should take is to establish an agreement, a set of guidelines for safe use of addictive medications (see appendix D for an example). This agreement describes the behavioral restrictions under which a patient can begin and continue to use opioids. In order to have a prescription renewed, the patient must live up to this code of behavior.

Patients and their doctors believe that such an agreement is a key to the safe prescribing and the safe use of these medications, because if patients take the medications within this code of behavior, they will protect themselves from misuse of the drugs. They won't take more medication than has been prescribed. Furthermore, they are unlikely to adopt any other aberrant or drug-seeking behaviors. Evidence of trouble or of addiction will arise if patients stray from that agreement, and if a problem does arise, a patient's medical team should recognize the problem early and take steps to address it.

Three Strikes

Many physicians who use opioid agreements with their patients have a "three strikes and you're out" policy. If a first violation occurs, the doctor will talk with the patient and let him or her know that the medical team is completely serious about the rules. A first strike is usually not cause for serious alarm; people do make innocent mistakes, such as losing a prescription and needing an earlier refill as a result. If a second strike comes closely on the heels of the first, that's an indication that using these medications may be a problem. At this point, the medical team will have a very blunt conversation with the patient. Simply put, a third strike will mean that the patient will no longer receive prescriptions for the medication involved.

Pseudoaddiction

Tara, in her early fifties, had a number of surgeries on her ankle to repair damage caused by repeated sprains. The pain medicine prescribed by her doctor had been relieving her pain fairly effectively, but not as much as she'd hoped. Then it began to worsen. The pain may have simply intensified, or she may have built up a tolerance for the medication she was using. For whatever reason, Tara has begun to take her medicine a bit more often than prescribed, and she has run out of her medication early. She had not taken excessive doses, experienced any level of euphoria, or showed any behavioral or physical effects of drug-abusing behavior. From Tara's physician's perspective, it might seem that Tara was abusing her medication because she was making repeated phone calls for refills earlier than expected.

In such cases, a physician may easily assume that drug abuse is occurring. Some in the medical field call this *pseudoaddiction*. This term is misleading, however, because it implies that an addiction problem of some sort is occurring. But that's not necessarily the case. Before her physician concludes that Tara was abusing medication, he or she should first determine whether a change in medication, dosage, frequency, or route of delivery is needed for optimal pain relief. Tara should not have changed her own dosage or frequency without discussing it with her doctor. Her best option now is to talk with her doctor and carefully look at all her options. More medication might be advisable, but her doctor might also recommend that she explore some behavioral or psychological therapies. Whatever steps are taken should be in collaboration with a doctor.

Do not take matters into your own hands by simply taking more of the medication. If it isn't working as well as you expected, or as well as it had initially, that is not a reason to take higher or more frequent dosages than prescribed, *especially* if you have had a history of alcoholism or drug addiction.

Determining Appropriate Dose

Once patients sign the opioid agreement, the medical team works to determine the appropriate balance between the drug's beneficial and negative effects. The goal is to gain as much pain relief and functional improvement as possible *without* bringing on excessive side effects. The team will look at both the decrease in magnitude of pain—one of the key goals, of course—and at functional outcomes. For example, is the patient able to participate in more activities, like returning to work or participating in more social activities with friends? Once again, the medical team wants to see specific functional improvement as well as a decrease in pain intensity.

Evaluating Effectiveness

Starting an opioid medication is not an irreversible decision. The medication can be stopped if it isn't useful or causes too many side effects or behavioral problems. After an effective dose of the medication has been determined, patients can then make an informed decision about whether this is a course of action they want to follow. How bad are the side effects? How much pain relief are they getting? Is their overall quality of life better than it was without the drugs? Most people are able to make this decision fairly quickly because whether the medications are worth the effort and have the effect they want become obvious fairly quickly. Some may find that the side effects outweigh the drug's benefits. If the decision to discontinue opioid use is made, the medical team will taper the dose and take the patient off the drug. By tapering the medication over a period of one to two weeks, the problems of withdrawal are avoided.

On the other hand, if the patient and the health care team agree that he or she is functioning better and that it makes sense to keep taking the opioid, the doctor should feel comfortable continuing to prescribe it within these behavioral constraints. As patients demonstrate responsible use of this drug, doctors can, and often do, let a previous "strike" expire over time. Everybody's human, and from time to time, people are going to lose a prescription or have some other problem. Initially, however, the behavioral constraints must be very tight.

When Using Opioids, Don't Isolate Yourself

Once again, we want to emphasize the importance of keeping others—your sponsor, your AA or NA meeting, your family and friends—aware of your medical care and your use of opioids. Staying silent about your medication, no matter how innocent the reason, can set you on a course that may threaten your recovery.

Keep others in your life aware of what you're doing. They need to know your plan as you start your medical treatment with opioids, and you need to stay in touch as the days, weeks, and even months pass, regularly letting them know how you're managing. Remember, too, how valuable support groups can be. It's also important to talk with some trusted and objective person, be it your doctor, a loved one, or a friend who's in recovery. In isolation lies weakness; in connection with others, you'll find strength and safety.

In conclusion, under some circumstances it may be appropriate and safe for a person in recovery to use addictive medications, including opioids, for pain. Under the close supervision of a doctor and within the context of a plan complete with goals, rules, and expectations for safe use, the risks can be decreased to an acceptable level. After an evaluation period, the decision to continue taking addictive medications is based on the benefits achieved from the pain relief as judged by improved activity, rehabilitation, and quality of life.

Definitions

acetaminophen (uh-seet-uh-ME-no-fen). An over-the-counter nonaspirin medication that relieves pain and reduces fever. Occurs in combination with many medications.

acetylsalicylic acid (ASA) (uh-SE-til-sal-uh-SIL-ik acid). The chemical name for aspirin (see page 168).

acute pain. Pain that occurs immediately after illness or injury and resolves after healing.

addiction. An illness in which a person seeks and consumes a substance, such as alcohol, tobacco, or other drug, despite the fact that it causes harm.

allodynia (al-o-DIN-e-uh). An altered sensation in which normally nonpainful events are felt as being painful.

amino acid. Small molecules that are the building blocks of proteins.

analgesic (an-ul-JE-zik). A medication or agent that reduces pain.

anesthetic. A substance used to eliminate sensation.

antiseizure medication. A drug used to prevent seizures. Some of these drugs are effective in reducing pain that originates from a damaged nerve (neuropathic pain). Also called anti-epileptic or anticonvulsant medication.

aspirin. An over-the-counter medication that relieves pain, reduces inflammation, and reduces fever. It also reduces blood clotting, which can aggravate bleeding.

autonomic nervous system. The portion of the nervous system that regulates involuntary body functions, including those of the heart and intestine. Controls blood flow, digestion, and temperature regulation.

blood sedimentation test. A test that measures the speed (rate) at which red blood cells settle at the bottom of a column of blood in a glass tube. The rate depends on the amount of certain proteins in the blood. Elevated levels may indicate some types of inflammatory or infectious disorders. Also called erythrocyte sedimentation rate and sed rate.

bone scan. A test using a radioactive agent to identify injured, damaged, or diseased areas of bone. Often used to identify fractures or tumors that may not be visible on an X-ray.

botanical. See herb. "Botanical" is a synonym for "herb."

bursa. A fluid-containing sac near a joint or bony prominence that reduces friction between a tendon and a bone, or between bone and skin during movement.

celiac plexus (SE-le-ak PLEK-sus). A network of nerve fibers in the abdomen that conduct pain sensation from the abdominal organs, such as the liver, spleen, stomach, and pancreas.

cerebral cortex. Surface layer of the cerebrum. This part of the brain is involved in many of the higher functions, such as interpretation of sensory information, planning, and voluntary movement.

chronic pain. Pain that persists beyond the time of normal healing and can last from a few months to many years. Can result from disease, such as arthritis, or from an injury or surgery. Also can occur without a known injury or disease.

clinical trials. Research studies in which a treatment or therapy is tested in people to see whether it is safe and effective.

computed tomography. An X-ray technique that uses a computer to construct cross-sectional images of the body. Also called CT scan and formerly known as CAT scan.

corticosteroids. Anti-inflammatory drugs created from or based on a naturally occurring hormone produced by the cortex of the adrenal glands (cortisone).

cortisone. A naturally occurring hormone produced by the cortex of the adrenal glands. It decreases inflammation.

COX-2 inhibitor. A nonsteroidal anti-inflammatory drug (NSAID) that specifically inhibits an enzyme known as cyclo-oxygenase-2 (COX-2), which contributes to inflammation. These drugs are used to treat pain and may be less likely to cause gastrointestinal bleeding than other NSAIDs.

depression. An illness that involves the body, mood, and thoughts. The symptoms of depression often include feelings of sadness, hopelessness, or pessimism, and changes in sleep, appetite, and thinking.

electromyography (EMG). A test to evaluate the function of nerves and muscles and to detect disease or injury to either.

endorphins. Naturally occurring molecules made up of amino acids. Endorphins attach to special receptors in the brain and spinal cord to stop pain messages. These are the same receptors that respond to morphine and other opioid analgesics.

enkephalins (en-KEF-uh-lins). Naturally occurring molecules in the brain. Enkephalins attach to special receptors in your brain and spinal cord to stop pain messages. They also affect other functions within the brain and nervous system. These are the same receptors that respond to morphine and other opioid analgesics.

enzymes. Proteins that speed up and regulate chemical reactions in the body.

epidural anesthesia. A form of regional anesthesia where local anesthetic is injected into the epidural space (near the spinal cord, but not in the cerebrospinal fluid). It is used for labor analgesia, as well as for abdominal, pelvic, and lower extremity surgery. When the medication is given through a catheter, it can provide postoperative pain relief for a variety of surgeries from the neck down.

epidural steroid injection. Injection of anti-inflammatory medication (steroid or cortisone) into the epidural space. Used to relieve pain caused by a "pinched nerve" or "slipped disk."

facet joint (FAS-ut joint). A joint between two adjacent vertebrae. Adjacent vertebrae are connected by the intervertebral disk in the front and two facet joints in the back.

field block injection. A procedure used to relax a muscle or to reduce muscle pain and inflammation. The targeted muscle is injected with a local anesthetic and corticosteroid.

general anesthesia. A controlled state of unawareness, induced by an injected or inhaled medication, that renders a patient unconscious and unresponsive to surgical pain.

glandulars. Dietary ingredients or supplements that are made from the glands of animals.

heavy metals. A class of metals that, in chemical terms, have a density at least five times that of water. They are widely used in industry. A few examples of heavy metals that are toxic and have contaminated some dietary supplements are lead, arsenic, and mercury.

herb. A plant or plant part that is used for its flavor, scent, and/or therapeutic properties.

intraspinal. Within or into the vertebral column, which contains the epidural space, spinal cord, and cerebrospinal fluid.

intravenous. Within or into a vein.

limbic system. The portion of the brain that produces emotions.

local anesthetic. A medication that blocks pain nerve signals, movement nerve signals, or both in a specific part of the body.

magnetic resonance imaging (MRI). An image produced by use of magnetic fields and radio waves to visualize body structures.

myofascial pain. Pain and tenderness in the muscles and adjacent fibrous tissue (fascia).

narcotics. A group of drugs that cause sleepiness. These drugs include the opioids (morphine and its derivatives), which relieve pain by preventing transmission of pain messages to the brain. Narcotics also refers to a classification of controlled substances that includes LSD, marijuana, and cocaine, which are not opioids.

nerve block. An injection of local anesthetic around a nerve, preventing pain messages traveling along that nerve pathway from reaching the brain. Nerve blocks can also prevent movement signals from reaching muscles, causing weakness or temporary paralysis. Used most often to relieve pain for a short period, such as during a surgery.

neurolytic. A substance or procedure that destroys nerves to relieve pain.

neuropathic pain. Pain that originates from a damaged nerve or nervous system.

nociceptors (no-sih-SEP-turs). Nerve endings that are attached to peripheral nerves that detect potential or actual tissue damage. They sense unpleasant situations such as extreme heat, cold, a cut, or pressure.

nonsteroidal anti-inflammatory drugs (NSAIDs, or "en-SAIDS"). Medications, used to reduce inflammation, that are not corticosteroid-based. These medications inhibit cyclooxygenase (COX-1 and COX-2), which contributes to inflammation. See also COX-2 inhibitor.

opioids. Prescription medications, like morphine, that relieve pain by binding to receptors in the brain and spinal cord. Some are natural compounds derived from opium, called opiates, and others are synthetic medications that work in a similar way.

oral. Of or by the mouth.

pain. An unpleasant sensory and emotional experience associated with actual or potential tissue damage, or described in terms of such damage.

pain center. A facility with a group of physicians and other health care professionals whose collective expertise allows for the management of a variety of pain problems.

pain clinic. A facility with one or more physicians and other health care professionals who specialize in the treatment of painful conditions, such as back pain or headaches.

pain pump. A device that is surgically implanted in the lower abdomen, where it provides a steady stream of medication—typically an opioid—to the cerebrospinal fluid.

pain rehabilitation program. A program that provides comprehensive, rehabilitative therapy for people suffering from chronic pain.

pain scale. A system of rating pain. Often based on a scale of 0 to 10, with 0 being no pain and 10 being the worst imaginable pain.

pain threshold. The point (intensity) at which a sensation becomes painful.

pain tolerance level. The amount of pain that a person can endure and remain functional.

patient controlled analgesia (PCA). A system that allows patients to control the amount of pain medicine they receive. The patient pushes a button and a machine delivers a dose of pain medicine into the bloodstream through a vein.

peer reviewed. Reviewed before publication by a group of experts in the same field.

peripheral nerves. Nerves that run from the spinal cord to all other parts of the body. They transmit messages from the spinal cord and the brain to and from other parts of the body and send sensory signals back to the spinal cord and brain.

phantom pain. Pain or discomfort following amputation that feels as if it originates from the missing limb.

physical dependence. The physical condition in which rapid discontinuation of a substance, such as alcohol, tobacco, or a drug, causes a withdrawal reaction.

rebound pain. The result of intermittent use of a pain medication, which makes a person's pain worse because of changing medication levels. It is most typical of headaches.

regional anesthesia. A form of surgical anesthesia in which specific regions of the body are rendered insensitive to surgical pain, without altering consciousness. Regional anesthesia is often combined with sedation to relieve anxiety during surgery.

selective serotonin reuptake inhibitors (SSRIs). Medications used to relieve depression. They may work by increasing the availability of a brain chemical (serotonin) that helps to regulate mood.

serotonin (ser-oh-TOE-nin). A brain chemical (neurotransmitter) that helps to regulate mood. A lack of it may lead to depression.

side effects. Unwanted changes produced by medication or other treatment, ranging from minor and temporary, such as dry mouth, to more serious, such as gastrointestinal bleeding.

spinal. Referring to the spine. Also means a form of regional anesthesia where local anesthetic is injected into the cerebrospinal fluid. It is often used for abdominal, pelvic, or lower extremity surgery.

spinal cord. The bundle of nerves that extends from the base of the brain to the small of the back. It processes information and conducts impulses between the brain and the rest of the body.

spinal cord stimulator. A device intended to relieve chronic pain. The spinal cord is electrically stimulated so that a new sensation, such as tingling, overrides the pain sensation.

stellate ganglion block. A procedure designed to relieve pain that is caused by overactivity of the sympathetic nervous system in the upper extremities, the head, or the neck. A local anesthetic is injected into the front of the neck to block sympathetic nerves without blocking sensory pathways.

substance P. A protein substance that stimulates nerve endings at an injury site and within the spinal cord, increasing pain messages.

sympathetic nerve block. An injection of an anesthetic to relieve pain resulting from abnormal activity of the sympathetic nervous system. The sympathetic nerves control circulation and perspiration and are part of the autonomic nervous system.

testimonials. Information provided by individuals who claim to have been helped or cured by a particular product. The information provided lacks the necessary elements to be evaluated in a rigorous and scientific manner and is not used in the scientific literature.

thalamus. A portion of the brain that relays impulses, including sensory information from the sensory nerves. Sensory nerves enable people to feel objects that they touch and allow people to feel pain.

tolerance. The process by which a person adapts to a specific substance, so larger amounts of the prescribed medication or a new medication is needed to achieve the same results.

topical agents. Medications that are applied to the skin rather than ingested or injected. They can come in the form of a cream or a gel. Also called ointments.

transdermal. Entering via the skin, such as a medicated lotion being absorbed through the skin.

tricyclic antidepressants. A group of drugs used to relieve symptoms of depression. These drugs may also help relieve pain.

trigger point. Places on the body where muscles and adjacent fibrous tissue (fascia) are sensitive to touch. These areas are generally in the upper and lower back muscles, but they may occur elsewhere.

withdrawal. The physical or psychological state experienced when certain substances or medications are discontinued rapidly.

X-ray. Electromagnetic waves of short wavelength that penetrate most matter and can produce an image on film.

APPENDIX B: Common Pain Medications:
Safe / Caution / Danger

These pain medications are grouped by their relative abuse potential and risk to patients in recovery. While such risks have not been fully analyzed in medical research, clinical experience suggests these categories as a starting point for examining risk.

> **GREEN:** *Safe*
> Little risk of relapse. However, these medicines can still cause problems. For example, an overdose of acetaminophen can cause fatal liver damage.

acetaminophen
Acular
Advil
Aleve
amitriptyline
amoxapine
Anafranil
Anaprox
Ansaid
antipyrine /
   benzocaine /
   glycerin
aspirin
aspirin / calcium
   carbonate /
   magnesium
bupropion
Buspar
buspirone
capsaicin
carbamazepine
Cataflam
celecoxib

Celexa
citalopram
Clinoril
clomipramine
Cymbalta
Daypro
Depakene
Depakote
desipramine
diclofenac
diflunisal
Dilantin
divalproate
   sodium
Dolobid
doxepin
duloxetine
Elavil
escitalopram
etodolac
Feldene
fenoprofen
fluoxetine

flurbiprofen
fluvoxamine
gabapentin
Gabitril
ibuprofen
imipramine
Indocin
indomethacin
ketoprofen
ketorolac
Lamictal
lamotrigine
Lexapro
Lodine
maprotiline
meclofenamate
meloxicam
mirtazapine
Mobic
Motrin
nabumetone
Naprosyn
naproxen
nefazodone
Neurontin
Norpramin
nortriptyline
olanzapine
olanzapine /
   fluoxetine
Orudis
oxaprozin

oxycarbazepine
Pamelor
paroxetine
Paxil
phenytoin
piroxicam
protriptyline
Prozac
Relafen
Remeron
salsalate
sertraline
Sinequan
sulindac
Surmontil
Tegretol
tiagabine
Tofranil
tolmetin
Topamax
topiramate
Toradol
trazodone
Trileptal
trimipramine
Tylenol
valproic acid
venlafaxine
Vivactil
Zoloft
zonisamide

Some medications are listed more than once, by both generic and trade names. For example, the generic drug acetaminophen (note the small letter "a") is also known by the trade name Tylenol (capital "T"), among others. Both appear alphabetically in the "Green" column. If you can't find a medication here, ask your doctor or pharmacist for its generic name.

YELLOW: *Caution*		
Higher risk for patients in recovery: can be misused for intoxication and have potential for addiction. Should not be used as a first-line treatment, but may be a better choice than the medications listed on page 180. *Starred medications * require extra caution.	Ambien Amidone * Buprenex * * buprenorphine * * buprenorphine / naloxone * * butorphanol * Dolophine * Duragesic (patch) * * fentanyl (patch) * * methadone *	* Methadose * * nalbuphine * * Nubain * * Stadol * * Stadol NS * * Suboxone * * Subutex * tramadol tramadol / acetaminophen Ultracet Ultram ziconotide zolpidem

Categorization can be difficult in some cases. Butorphanol (Yellow), for example, is rarely used on the street by opioid addicts, but it does pose a risk for abuse and addiction—especially for health care professionals. Buprenorphine and methadone (Yellow, but starred for extra caution) are used as maintenance therapies for opioid addiction, yet also have abuse potential themselves. Fentanyl (Red), a highly addictive opioid, may be more safely used as a patch (Duragesic); however, some addicts apply several patches or even try to inject the gel intravenously—a very dangerous practice.

> **RED:** *Danger*
> High abuse or relapse potential. These should not be used as a first-line treatment. You and your doctor must follow all the guidelines in chapter 8 of this book.

Actiq
Alfenta
alfentanil
alprazolam
Anexsia
aspirin /
  caffeine /
  butalbital
Ativan
butalbital
chlordi-
  azepoxide
clidinium /
  chlordi-
  azepoxide
clonazepam
clorazepate
codeine
codeine /
  acetaminophen
codeine /
  promethazine
codeine
  phosphate
codeine sulfate
Compal
Dalmane
Darvocet
Darvon
Demerol

diazepam
dihydrocodeine /
  aspirin /
  caffeine
dihydrocodeine
  bitartrate /
  acetaminophen
  / caffeine
dihydromorphi-
  none
Dilaudid
Equagesic
Equanil
fentanyl
fentanyl citrate
fentanyl /
  droperidol
flurazepam
guaifenesin /
  codeine
  phosphate
Halcion
Hycodan
hydrocodone /
  acetaminophen
hydromorphone
Innovar
Kadian
Klonipin
Levo-Dromoran

levorphanol
Libritabs
Librium
Limbitrol
lorazepam
Lortab
Mepergan
meperidine
meprobamate
midazolam
Miltown
morphine
morphine /
  opium
morphine
  sulfate
MS Contin
Numorphan
opium
opium /
  belladona
  alkaloids
opium /
  paregoric
opium / tincture
oxazepam
oxycodone
oxycodone /
  acetaminophen
oxycodone /
  aspirin
OxyContin
oxymorphone
pentazocine
pentazocine /
  acetaminophen
pentazocine /
  naloxone
Percocet
Percodan

pethidine
promethazine /
  phenyl-
  ephrine /
  codeine
propoxyphene
propoxyphene
  napsulate /
  acetaminophen
remifentanil
Restoril
Roxicet
Roxicodone
Serax
Sonata
Sublimaze
Sufenta
Sufentanil
Synalgos-DC
Talacen
Talwin
Talwin
  Compound
Talwin NX
TC#3
temazepam
Tranxene
triazolam
Tussend
Tussionex
Tylenol with
  codeine
Tylox
Ultiva
Valium
Valrelease
Versed
Vicodin
Xanax
zaleplon

APPENDIX C

Keeping a Journal

As you learn techniques to manage your pain, you should see
an increase in your activity level and, perhaps, a decrease in
your pain level. A daily journal can help you track your
progress and determine the therapies or activities that seem to
be helping you the most. A journal is also a way to track the
goals you want to achieve and your progress in reaching them.

Many people think that their pain isn't influenced by factors such as work, stress, sleep, or physical activity. But after
a few months of tracking their pain levels and their activities,
they begin to notice some common patterns.

In addition, a journal can be a good way to express your
feelings about your pain or about other events that are happening in your life. Writing your thoughts and feelings on
paper can help you organize and sort through problems and
emotions and get them off your chest, similar to the way you
feel after a good heart-to-heart visit with a good friend or family member.

Pain level and activities

Health care professionals typically measure pain on a scale of
0 to 10, with 0 being no pain and 10 being the worst pain

imaginable. Use this scale as your guide by rating your pain level three times a day and recording it in your journal. In addition, briefly note what you were doing at that time of day. You can do this whenever it's convenient, but keep the times consistent. Many people choose to record their pain level in the morning when they wake up, after lunch, and in the evening before bed.

Use this scale as a guide when determining your level of pain.

0-1	2 to 3	3 to 4	5 to 6	7 to 8	8 to 9	10
no pain	mild pain	discomforting pain	distressing, moderate pain	severe pain	intense, very severe pain	worst pain imaginable

Keeping a log of your pain levels and activities allows you to:

Learn your pain pattern. Most people find that the changes in their pain levels are quite consistent. For example, your pain may generally be at its lowest level in the morning and at its highest level in the evening. Recording your pain levels helps you determine your pain pattern.

Link your pain with your activities. If your pain is always the worst in the evening, for example, try to determine the reason. See if certain activities seem to correlate with an increase or a decrease in your pain level. Are you sitting or standing too long? Is your rush to get dinner ready a contributing factor? Or perhaps you're just tired?

Identify flares. Recording your pain levels helps draw attention to inconsistencies. If your pain level at noon is normally a 3, and then one day it's a 6, noting the difference may prompt you to think about your morning. Did you do something differently? Did you have a particularly stressful morning?

See your progress. If you feel you aren't making progress, reading your journal can help you realize that your life has improved, even though the process may seem slow. Your journal can also give you clues about why some areas remain difficult.

Mood

On a scale of 0 to 10, with 0 being poor and 10 being excellent, rate your mood. This exercise can help you see that even though your pain and your mood are closely aligned, they aren't linked together. Typically, the worse your pain, the worse your mood, and vice versa. However, as you begin to feel more in control of your pain, you may find your mood improving at a faster rate than the improvement in your pain levels. Rating your mood can also help you see that even though you may not be able to eliminate your pain, you can learn to live with it and still be happy.

Sleep

A good night's sleep better equips you to handle your day. However, getting enough sleep can be difficult because your pain may keep you up at night. In contrast, some people spend too much time in bed. This can also reduce your pain tolerance. Once a day, record how many hours you slept during the past twenty-four hours. Eight hours is average, but the amount of sleep each person needs varies. Your goal should be to feel rested when you wake up.

A Sample Journal Page

Date: _____ Hours slept: _____

	7 a.m.	1 p.m.	10 p.m.
Pain level:	_____	_____	_____
Mood:	_____	_____	_____
Activity:	_____	_____	_____

Comments:

Guidelines for Safely Taking Addictive Medications

There may be a risk of physical dependence or tolerance with long-term use of controlled substances such as opioids (narcotic analgesics), benzodiazepine tranquilizers, and barbiturate sedatives.

Because these prescribed controlled substances have the potential for physical dependence, tolerance, or addiction, your doctor needs to make sure that these medications are properly prescribed and patients are educated to use them correctly.

Before you receive your first prescription for a controlled substance, your health care provider should establish guidelines for their safe use. You are expected to follow these guidelines for both initial and continued prescription of controlled substances. Here are some typical guidelines:

- All controlled substances must be prescribed by one health care provider. Initially this source can be a specialist. However, after you are on a stable dose, it may be possible for your primary care provider to assume responsibility for prescribing these medications.

- All controlled substances should be bought at the same pharmacy, if at all possible.
- Tell your health care provider immediately if you start to take any new medications, if you have new medical conditions, or if you have any side effects.
- You must authorize your health care provider to discuss all tests, lab results, and other diagnostic and treatment details with other professionals who give you health care.
- You may not share, sell, or give these medications to others.
- Do not stop these medications abruptly. This could cause serious side effects or withdrawal
- Random (unannounced) urine or blood tests may be requested, and your cooperation is required. If unauthorized medications are found, or if the prescribed medications are not found, you will be in violation of the agreement.
- You must be careful with your medication and prescription. Do not leave them where others might see them or have access to them.
- Bring the original containers of medications to each office visit.
- Since these medications may be dangerous to a person who is not used to their effects, especially a child, be sure to keep them safely out of reach.
- Prescriptions or medications may not be replaced if they are lost, get wet, are destroyed, are left on an airplane, and so forth. If your medication has been

stolen and you complete a police report regarding the theft, an exception may be possible.

• Early refills generally are not given. A prescription for an early refill may be given if you or your health care provider will be out of town when a refill is due. These prescriptions instruct the pharmacist not to refill them before the appropriate date.

• You will give all clinicians who are involved in your health care permission to share medical information about you. In addition to your pain physician, this includes other specialists, emergency room physicians, and pharmacists. You may have to contact each provider separately to provide this permission.

• Failure to comply with these policies may result in your health care provider's decision to stop prescribing opioids or other medications.

• Your prescription will not be renewed if you do not keep your scheduled appointments.

• Any medication treatment is initially a trial. Continuation of the medication is based on evidence of benefit.

• You should request medication refills one week before the renewal date. Do not phone for prescriptions after business hours or on weekends.

Resources for Traditional and Complementary Medicine

CAM (Complementary and Alternative Medicine) on PubMed

Web site: www.nlm.nih.gov/nccam/camonpubmed.html

CAM on PubMed is an Internet database developed jointly by the National Center for Complementary and Alternative Medicine (NCCAM) and the National Library of Medicine (NLM). It contains bibliographic citations to articles on complementary and alternative medicine in scientifically based, peer-reviewed journals. These citations are a subset of the NLM's PubMed system, which contains more than 12 million journal citations from the MEDLINE database and additional life science journals important to health researchers, practitioners, and consumers. CAM on PubMed displays links to publisher Web sites; some sites offer the full text of articles.

Cochrane Library

Web site: www.cochrane.org

The Cochrane Library is a collection of science-based reviews from the Cochrane Collaboration, an international nonprofit organization that seeks to provide "up-to-date, accurate

information about the effects of health care." Its authors analyze the results of rigorous clinical trials (research studies with
people) on a given topic and prepare summaries called sys-
tematic reviews. Abstracts, or brief summaries, of these reviews can be read online without charge. You can search by
treatment name, such as the name of an herb, or by medical
condition. Fee-based subscriptions to the full text are offered
and are carried by some libraries.

Federal Trade Commission (FTC)

Web site: www.ftc.gov
Toll-free phone: 1-877-FTC-HELP (1-877-382-4357)
The FTC works for the consumer to prevent fraudulent, deceptive, and unfair business practices in the marketplace and
to provide information to help consumers spot, stop, and
avoid them. To file a complaint or to get free information on
consumer issues, call toll-free 1-877-FTC-HELP, or use the online complaint form found at www.ftc.gov. Consumers who
want to learn how to recognize fraudulent or unproven health
care products and services can find information at www
.ftc.gov/cureall.

National Center for Complementary and Alternative Medicine (NCCAM) Clearinghouse

Web site: nccam.nih.gov
Toll-free phone in the U.S.: 1-888-644-6226
International phone: 301-519-3153
E-mail: info@nccam.nih.gov
TTY (for deaf or hard-of-hearing callers): 1-866-464-3615
Fax: 1-866-464-3616
Fax-on-demand service: 1-888-644-6226

Address: NCCAM Clearinghouse, P.O. Box 7923, Gaithersburg, MD 20898-7923
The Clearinghouse provides information on NCCAM and topics in complementary and alternative medicine. Services include fact sheets, other publications, and searches of federal databases of scientific and medical literature.

National Institutes of Health (NIH) Office of Dietary Supplements (ODS)

Web site: ods.od.nih.gov
E-mail: ods@nih.gov
Phone: 301-435-2920
Fax: 301-480-1845
Address: 6100 Executive Blvd., Bethesda, MD 20892-7517
The mission of ODS is to explore the potential role of dietary supplements to improve health care. It promotes the scientific study of dietary supplements through conducting and coordinating scientific research and compiling and disseminating research results. ODS provides all its public information through its Web site, including the International Bibliographic Information on Dietary Supplements (IBIDS) database containing abstracts of peer-reviewed scientific literature at ods.od.nih.gov/databases/ibids.html.

National Library of Medicine (NLM)

Web site: www.nlm.nih.gov
Toll-free phone: 1-888-346-3656
E-mail: custserv@nlm.nih.gov
Fax: 301-402-1384
Address: 8600 Rockville Pike, Bethesda, MD 20894
NLM is the world's largest medical library. Services include

MEDLINE, NLM's premier bibliographic database covering the fields of medicine, nursing, dentistry, veterinary medicine, the health care system, and preclinical science. MEDLINE contains indexed journal citations and abstracts from more than 4,600 journals published in the United States and more than seventy other countries. MEDLINE is accessible through NLM's PubMed system at pubmed.gov. NLM also maintains DIRLINE (dirline.nlm.nih.gov), a database that contains locations and descriptive information about a variety of health organizations, including those for complementary and alternative medicine.

U.S. Food and Drug Administration (FDA)

Web site: www.fda.gov
Toll-free phone: 1-888-INFO-FDA (1-888-463-6332)
Address: 5600 Fishers Lane, Rockville, MD 20857-0001
The FDA's mission is to promote and protect the public health by helping safe and effective products reach the market in a timely way, and by monitoring products for continued safety after they are in use. Its Web site information includes "Tips for the Savvy Supplement User: Making Informed Decisions and Evaluating Information" (www.cfsan.fda.gov/~dms/ds -savvy.html) and updated safety information on supplements (www.cfsan.fda.gov/~dms/ds-warn.html).

To report serious adverse events or illnesses related to FDA-regulated products, such as drugs, medical devices, medical foods, and dietary supplements, contact MedWatch through its Web site (www.fda.gov/medwatch/report/consumer/ consumer.htm), toll-free phone (1-800-FDA-1088), or fax (1-800-FDA-0178).

To report a general complaint or concern about food products, including dietary supplements, you may contact the consumer complaint coordinator at the FDA district office nearest you. To find that office's phone number, visit www .fda.gov/opacom/backgrounders/complain.html, or check the government listings in your telephone book.

The Twelve Steps of Alcoholics Anonymous

1. We admitted we were powerless over alcohol—that our lives had become unmanageable.
2. Came to believe that a Power greater than ourselves could restore us to sanity.
3. Made a decision to turn our will and our lives over to the care of God *as we understood Him*.
4. Made a searching and fearless moral inventory of ourselves.
5. Admitted to God, to ourselves, and to another human being the exact nature of our wrongs.
6. Were entirely ready to have God remove all these defects of character.
7. Humbly asked Him to remove our shortcomings.
8. Made a list of all persons we had harmed, and became willing to make amends to them all.
9. Made direct amends to such people wherever possible, except when to do so would injure them or others.
10. Continued to take personal inventory and when we were wrong promptly admitted it.

11. Sought through prayer and meditation to improve our conscious contact with God *as we understood Him,* praying only for knowledge of His will for us and the power to carry that out.
12. Having had a spiritual awakening as the result of these steps, we tried to carry this message to alcoholics, and to practice these principles in all our affairs.

The Twelve Steps of AA are taken from *Alcoholics Anonymous,* 4th ed. (New York: Alcoholics Anonymous World Services, Inc., 2001), 59–60.

Notes

Chapter 1: What Is Pain?

1. From "Economic Impact of Back Pain Substantial," a Duke University study published Jan. 1, 2004, in the journal *Spine* and at dukemednews.dukc.cdu/news/article.php?id−7312.

2. American Chiropractic Association, "Back Pain Statistics," www.amerchiro.org/media/whatis/benefits.shtml.

3. National Institute of Neurological Disorders and Stroke, "Hope through Research," www.ninds.nih.gov.

4. American Cancer Society, "Cancer Statistics 2005," www.cancer .org/docroot/med/content/med_2_1X_cancer_statistics_2005.asp.

5. H. Merskey, ed., "Classification of Chronic Pain: Description of Chronic Pain Syndromes and Definitions of Pain Terms," *Pain,* Suppl 3 (1986): S217.

Chapter 2: Types of Pain

1. Jeremy Rome, ed. in chief, *Mayo Clinic on Chronic Pain,* 2nd ed. (Rochester, MN: Mayo Foundation for Medical Education and Research, 2002), 10.

Chapter 3: Addiction and Its Treatments

1. Alan I. Leshner, *Understanding Drug Addiction: Insights from the Research in Principles of Addiction Medicine* (Chevy Chase, MD: American Society of Addiction Medicine, 2003).

2. Marlene Oscar-Berman and Ksenija Marinkovic, "Alcoholism and the Brain: An Overview," available on National Institute on Alcohol Abuse and Alcoholism Web site, www.niaaa.nih.gov/publications/arh27-2/125-133.htm.

3. Ibid.

4. Allan W. Graham, Terry K. Schultz, Michael Mayo-Smith, Richard K. Ries, and Bonnie B. Wilford, eds., *Principles of Addiction Medicine*, 3rd ed. (Chevy Chase, MD: American Society of Addiction Medicine, 2003), 47–56.

5. Lee N. Robins, "Vietnam Veterans' Rapid Recovery from Heroin Addiction: A Fluke or Normal Expectation?" *Addiction* 88 (1993): 1041–54.

6. "About A.A.," Alcoholics Anonymous Web site, www .alcoholics-anonymous.org.

7. Material on Narcotics Anonymous is adapted from its Web site, www.na.org.

Chapter 4: Pain Medications

1. *Mayo Clinic on Chronic Pain*, 57–59.

2. The following discussion of opioids is adapted from Drew Pinsky, Marvin D. Seppala, Robert J. Meyers, John Gardin, William White, and Stephanie Brown, *When Painkillers Become Dangerous: What Everyone Needs to Know about OxyContin and Other Prescription Drugs* (Center City, MN: Hazelden Foundation, 2004), 5–6.

Chapter 5: Considering Complementary Medicine for Pain

1. National Center for Complementary and Alternative Medicine, "More Than One-Third of U.S. Adults Use Complementary and Alternative Medicine, According to New Government Survey," www.nccam.nih.gov/news/2004/052704.htm.

2. S. K. Avants, A. Margolin, T. R. Holford, T. R. Kosten, "A Randomized Controlled Trial of Auricular Acupuncture for Cocaine Dependence," *Archives of Internal Medicine* 160 (15) (August 14/26, 2000): 2305–12.

3. Adapted from "My Potential: Biofeedback," www.mypotential
.ie/biofeedback/.

4. Adapted from National Center for Complementary and Alternative Medicine, "What Is Complementary and Alternative Medicine (CAM)?" www.nccam.nih.gov/health/whatiscam/ and other sources.

5. Ibid.

6. Cited on National Institutes of Health Web site; actual sources are S. W. Lazar, G. Bush, R. L. Gollub et al., "Functional Brain Mapping of the Relaxation Response and Meditation," *Neuroreport* 11 (7) (2000): 1581–85; and R. J. Davidson, J. Kabat-Zinn, J. Schumacher et al., "Alterations in Brain and Immune Function Produced by Mindfulness Meditation," *Psychosomatic Medicine* 65 (4) (2003): 564–70.

7. Adapted from National Center for Complementary and Alternative Medicine, "What Is Complementary and Alternative Medicine (CAM)?" www.nccam.nih.gov/health/whatiscam/.

8. Ibid.

9. Ibid.

10. Adapted from Christina Brown, *The Book of Yoga* (Bath, UK: Paragon Publishing, 2002).

11. Adapted from National Center for Complementary and Alternative Medicine, "Ten Things to Know about Evaluating Medical Resources on the Web," www.nccam.nih.gov/health/webresources/.

12. National Center for Complementary and Alternative Medicine, "Herbal Supplements: Consider Safety, Too," www.nccam.nih.gov/health/supplement-safety.

Chapter 6: Winning Ways to Cope with Pain

1. Material on deep breathing, progressive relaxation, and guided imagery is adapted from the University of South Florida Center for Human Development (USF), "Stress Reduction Techniques," usfweb2.usf.edu/counsel/SELF-HLP/stress_red.htm.

Index

About the Authors

Marvin D. Seppala, M.D., is chief medical officer at the Hazelden Foundation. Prior to working at Hazelden, Dr. Seppala was a psychiatric consultant at the Native American Rehabilitation Association in Portland, Oregon, and at Springbrook Northwest in Newberg, Oregon. Beginning in the 1980s, Dr. Seppala held a private practice and was a psychiatric consultant to several addiction treatment centers in the Portland, Oregon, and Minneapolis, Minnesota, areas. He is a member of the board of the American Society of Addiction Medicine and a founding member of the Oregon Society of Addiction Medicine. Dr. Seppala is author of *Clinician's Guide to the Twelve Step Principles* and co-author of *When Painkillers Become Dangerous.*

David P. Martin, M.D., Ph.D., is board certified in anesthesiology with advanced certification in pain medicine. Since 1993 he has been at the Mayo Clinic in Rochester, Minnesota, where he is a consultant in the Department of Anesthesiology and an assistant professor of anesthesiology at the Mayo Clinic College of Medicine. He earned his M.D. degree, and a Ph.D. in neuroscience, from Washington University School of Medicine in Saint Louis, Missouri.

Joseph Moriarity is a freelance writer living in Forest Lake, Minnesota. He writes extensively about health, medical care, chemical dependency and recovery, education, and the environment for organizations, magazines, journals, and newspapers.

Hazelden, a national nonprofit organization founded in 1949, helps people reclaim their lives from the disease of addiction. Built on decades of knowledge and experience, Hazelden offers a comprehensive approach to addiction that addresses the full range of patient, family, and professional needs, including treatment and continuing care for youth and adults, research, higher learning, public education and advocacy, and publishing.

A life of recovery is lived "one day at a time." Hazelden publications, both educational and inspirational, support and strengthen lifelong recovery. In 1954, Hazelden published *Twenty-Four Hours a Day,* the first daily meditation book for recovering alcoholics, and Hazelden continues to publish works to inspire and guide individuals in treatment and recovery, and their loved ones. Professionals who work to prevent and treat addiction also turn to Hazelden for evidence-based curricula, informational materials, and videos for use in schools, treatment programs, and correctional programs.

Through published works, Hazelden extends the reach of hope, encouragement, help, and support to individuals, families, and communities affected by addiction and related issues.

For questions about Hazelden publications, please call **800-328-9000** or visit us online at **hazelden.org/bookstore**.